Natural Dualism and Mental Disorder

This book presents an integrative, dualist model of mental disorder for psychiatry, as a counter to the so-called "biomedical" approach that dominates the field today. Starting with the humanist concept that mental disorder is real, it uses a computational approach to build a genuinely bio-psycho-social model. This shows that mental disorder is primarily psychological in nature, not biological.

The historical background extends as far as Descartes, and proceeds via some of the revolutionary thinkers who have shaped modern society. In particular, it builds on the work of George Boole, Alan Turing and Claude Shannon to construct a radically new concept of the mind as a real, informational space which, for better off for worse, can malfunction. It extends this idea to build models of personality, of personality disorder, and then of mental disorder. Finally, the concepts are tested against a variety of themes from other fields to show its generality.

Based in the philosophy of science and of mind, this work represents a radical departure from anything in the history of psychiatry. Its purpose is to provide a formal, articulated model of mental disorder to fill the theoretical void at the core of modern psychiatry. This book is written for medical students and recent graduates, for psychiatrists, psychologists, social workers and, broadly, anybody with an interest in human affairs, such as philosophy, politics and other related fields.

Niall McLaren is an Australian psychiatrist with lengthy experience in remote area psychiatry and in the application of the philosophy of science to psychiatry.

Natural Dualism and Mental Disorder

The Biocognitive Model in Psychiatry

Niall McLaren

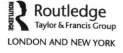

Routledge
Taylor & Francis Group

LONDON AND NEW YORK

First published 2022
by Routledge
2 Park Square, Milton Park, Abingdon, Oxon OX14 4RN

and by Routledge
605 Third Avenue, New York, NY 10158

Routledge is an imprint of the Taylor & Francis Group, an informa business

British Library Cataloguing-in-Publication Data
A catalog record has been requested for this book

ISBN: 978-1-032-02530-8 (hbk)
ISBN: 978-1-032-02532-2 (pbk)
ISBN: 978-1-003-18379-2 (ebk)

DOI: 10.4324/9781003183792

Typeset in Galliard
by MPS Limited, Dehradun

Contents

Figures

Tables

Preface

When I was aged 34, a senior consultant psychiatrist and head of department of psychiatry at the Veterans' Affairs Hospital, in Perth, Western Australia, I decided to go back to school. I had applied to work toward a PhD jointly in psychiatry and in philosophy but, because I had no undergraduate credits in philosophy, I had to enroll as a student to complete three units. I chose courses in the philosophy of mind, of science and of language. As I was working full-time and studying in other areas, as well as trying to lead a normal life, my course was spread over two years.

After twelve years of hard work, I was looking forward to being a carefree student again but... the first week back on campus was a shock. I had been placed in tutorials with second year (sophomore) students who had already completed Philosophy 100 and at least one other course. By the end of the first week, I was ready to withdraw. It was painfully clear to me that these ... kids, really, could think better than I could. Oh, the humiliation. But I persevered and survived, and it became a turning point in my life, except something unexpected happened.

The first part of the course on philosophy of language was a crash course in propositional logic, twelve lectures and twelve tutorials. That was fascinating but, by the end, it was becoming clear that the further I moved into the world of philosophy, the more distant I became from my psychiatric colleagues. Very quickly, I learned that pointing out any errors of logic in their reasoning was not a good move. To my surprise, they weren't grateful; at best, they were miffed but, more often, they became angry and stamped off. The reason was just that, in medical school, we weren't trained to think. Instead, we memorised vast quantities of material to serve back to the examiners on demand. From talking to today's medical students, it seems that nothing much has changed, or maybe it's even worse.

As a result, this book is probably unlike anything you've seen so far in your education. If you're a medical student, you will be familiar with large, heavy texts with lots of pictures, setting out the science of biology and the basic medical sciences, such as pathology, microbiology, pharmacology and so on. That's also likely to be true of fields such as psychology, nursing, physiotherapy and the other clinical specialties.

The essential point of these ponderous books is that if you learn them, you will pass your course. The texts contain all the material you need to know, neatly set out in entertaining style for you to memorise. If you're lucky, you may get a bit of history thrown in but, while each text presents the current state of empirical knowledge, most say very little as to how it got there. Everything is presented as fact, and all you have to do is absorb it to get ahead. The unstated corollary is that you are not invited to debate the material. If you're reading about, say, coronaviruses, the authors are the experts and you're the amateur, so just keep reading diligently and don't argue with what they tell you.

When it comes to psychiatry, you'll probably use a book that presents the information in much the same format, setting out the essentials of what the editors want you to know in digestible chunks. Again, you will not be invited to argue with the authorities. If they say that depression is a biological disease of the brain, and if you want to pass the course, that's what you must say. And that's exactly what psychiatric texts do say, in the same kindly but firm tones you heard in Biology 100.

What you won't be told is that there is actually no proof of that claim, that all the talk about neurotransmitters and single nucleotide polymorphisms found in genome-wide association studies doesn't belong to any articulated theory of mind or model of mental disorder. You may be told that it all fits with something called the biopsychosocial model, but you will never see a copy of it, and nobody will ever tell you what it models. Is it a model of mind? Or of mental disorder? Does it make predictions that lead to a formal research program?

Perhaps it would be better for your career if you didn't ask these questions. Unlike the rest of medicine, and the other fields mentioned above, psychiatry is unique in not having an articulated model of its field, mental disorder. It also doesn't have a theory or model of mind, or of personality, or of personality disorder. If you have already worked this out yourself, you'd better keep quiet about it as academic psychiatrists are rather touchy on this point. As a matter of established fact, what academic psychiatrists study and research and teach has none of the essential features of an empirical science, and all the features of an ideology. Perhaps there are fields where that doesn't matter so much but, when you are dealing with people's lives and freedom, as psychiatrists do, the absence of an intellectual structure is a very serious matter.

And herein lies the difference in this book: starting at the most elementary level, it assembles a formal, humanist model of mind, and thence of mind-body interaction. This is *a* solution to the mind-body problem; I am not claiming it is *the* solution to that ancient question but, as a model for psychiatry, it leads directly to a model of mental disorder. Along the way, it defines personality, and thence personality disorder. But it does so in a way you may find somewhat confusing, although students of mathematics and of philosophy will see it as more or less normal. As its foundation, it starts with some absolutely basic points, then elaborates on them to build a superstructure which I hope you will find convincing. You will be shown each step in the argument, with nothing presented as gospel, and leaving, I hope, no loose ends to bother you.

At the same time, the material covers a much broader range than is normal in medical education. There is a quite a bit of history, some potted biographies, chunks of philosophy, logic and fundamental mathematics, engineering, some neurophysiology, sociology, ethology, and even a section on economics. All this in about 75,000 words. Students who have reviewed it said they struggled a bit with some of the new concepts but soon found their feet, and enjoyed the experience of exploring new ideas, as distinct from being told what to think.

At the head of each chapter, you will find a brief summary of the points to be made, with a few recommendations for further reading at the end. There are not a lot of citations, partly because it is intended as a self-sufficient argument, not a distillation of the current state of knowledge, and partly because I refer to my previous work which does contain them.

It won't take much to realise I have my intellectual heroes, starting with the French polymath, René Descartes. Each of them was a bit odd in one way or another and, these days, would probably acquire half a dozen separate psychiatric diagnoses and a long list of powerful psychotropic drugs. And that would be the end of their creativity.

We can end with a quote from a memorable writer, Robert Youngson, from his entertaining book *Scientific Blunders*, which I strongly recommend:

> The whole history of science, right up to the present, is a story of refusal to accept fundamental new ideas; of determined adherence to the *status quo*; of the invention of acceptable explanations, however ridiculous, for uncomfortable facts; of older people of scientific eminence dying in confirmed possession of their life-long beliefs; and of painful readjustment of younger people to new concepts. (1998, p 293).

I hope your readjustment to the new concepts in this book comes as a relief, rather than painful.

Niall McLaren, Brisbane, Australia, January 2021

Part I
Basic principles

1 Setting the scene for natural dualism

You never change something by fighting the existing reality. To change something, build a new model that makes the existing model obsolete.
                                           Richard Buckminster Fuller (1895–1983)

The most that can be expected from any model is that it can supply a useful approximation to reality: All models are wrong; some models are useful.
                                                        George Box (1919–2013)

1.1 The psychiatric view. Monism and reductionism

In talking about mental disorder, we have to talk about mentality. These days, everybody accepts that there is a mind and that there are mental events which occur within that mental life. The only dispute relates to how to give a rational account of the mind: What is its nature? How does it come about? How does it interact with the body?

The simplest approach is *monism*, the idea that the universe is of a single or unitary nature. The most common view is that there is no more to the universe than the material realm of time and space, matter and energy, all governed by the laws of physics as we usually understand them. This means that ultimately, the mind is also physical in nature, that it is no different *in principle* from all other things that we can see, touch and measure. This concept is known as *materialist monism* or, more precisely, as *physicalism*. The other type of monism is that the universe is entirely mental in nature, better known as *idealism*. There is a further niche in the middle, *neutral monism*, which says that mind and material matter are both manifestations of a single substance which we haven't yet discovered. There are very few modern philosophers who would take either of the latter two views seriously so it seems physicalism wins by default *but...* there are serious problems with this option.

In a material universe, big things are built from smaller things, so the best way to understand the behaviour or properties of bigger things is to take them apart. As a form of explanation, *reductionism* says that the behaviour or properties of higher order entities are fully explained as functions of the behaviour or properties of the lower order entities of which they are composed. The whole of

DOI: 10.4324/9781003183792-1

modern western science is built upon this concept and, so far, it has served us very well.

Biological reductionism says that the appearance and behaviour of all life forms is fully explained by the actions of the chemicals that comprise the living organism. However, when this principle is applied to humans, it has to include the mind. Reductionism says that the whole of the human mental life, including properties of mind and all mental events without exception, can be fully explained as properties of the physical matter of the brain. It is an attempt to account for the phenomena of mind in physical terms, not least because any other option immediately bogs down in contradictions.

For a reductionist, a full account of the anatomy, physiology and genetics of the human brain will yield a full account of the mind in all its aspects, with no questions left unanswered. *Biological psychiatry* relies on materialist monism or physicalism for its theoretical basis. It says that all questions of mental disorder can be answered in their entirety by a full knowledge of brain pathology. In logical terms, knowledge of the brain is necessary and sufficient to explain mental disorder: there is nothing else that needs explaining, and there is nothing else that could be explanatory. This is how the experts see it:

- Psychiatric disorders are brain disorders... Psychiatric disorders *are* medical disorders [1] (David Kupfer, b. 1941, chairman of DSM5 Committee; emphasis in the original).
- First, the RDoC framework conceptualises mental illnesses as brain disorders... Second, (it) assumes that the dysfunction in neural circuits can be identified with the tools of (ordinary) neuroscience... [2] (Thomas Insel, b. 1951, former director of US NIMH, which disburses the great bulk of psychiatric research money in the US, ca. $1.5bln each year).

For psychiatrists, whose medical training is directly in the tradition of western materialist science, biological reductionism holds a powerful attraction as it appears to mesh neatly with the rest of biology, with no discontinuity. Absent reductionism, we would be forced to grapple with the idea of mental disorder being caused by errors in some sort of ghostly "thing" in the head, which definitely doesn't mesh with western science.[1]

Unfortunately for its supporters, no psychiatrist has ever offered a proof of biological reductionism, as McHugh and Slavney glumly observed:

> ... in contrast to cardiologists, psychiatrists cannot go directly from knowing the elements of the brain (neurons and synapses) to explaining the conscious

---

1 Reductionism has an additional appeal in that it allows people to embrace the concept of mental disorder while holding firm fundamentalist religious views. In that case, mental disorder is seen as nothing more than the body going wrong; the soul remains perfect, as when it was created.

experiences that are the essence of mental life. At the frontier of brain and mind, wherever that may be, the words we use change from tangibles (neurons and synapses) to intangibles (thoughts, moods, and perceptions) ... Unlike cardiologists, psychiatrists are unable to go directly from the molecular structure of a bodily organ to the functional results of that organ's action [3, p. 30].

There is indeed no such proof anywhere in the specialist literature of any field [4], meaning biological reductionism is wholly an ideological claim, divorced from scientific reality. The history of why it has become so influential is another story (see [5] for a very readable account of the history of biological psychiatry) but the narrative of a biological psychiatry has now become immune to, and, all too often, vehemently protected from, criticism, as philosopher Daniel Stoljar (b. 1967) noted:

The first thing to say when considering the truth of physicalism is that we live in an overwhelmingly physicalist or materialist intellectual culture. The result is that, as things currently stand, the standards of argumentation required to persuade someone of the truth of physicalism are much lower than the standards required to persuade someone of its negation [6].

Essentially, and not least because the alternatives seem so vague and uncertain, people *want* to believe that physicalism is the way to go, so they have never bothered too much about the details.

In a careful analysis of the concept, Stoljar considered three basic questions. If we say that everything is physical, firstly, what are we actually saying? Second, is it true? Third, what are the consequences of making this claim? He determined that physicalism is more an attitude than a consistent explanatory thesis. So, if we hear a noise from the roof at night, we assume it's amorous possums and not demons. If a friend ails, we don't automatically think of spells or possession states. And if his malady is depression, we assign it to the class of brain dysfunctions as a 'chemical imbalance of the brain.'

Guided by physicalism, we assume this because it sounds real, objective and amenable to intervention. As good rationalists, we don't want to resort to psychologism, i.e. to think of his depression as some indefinable hangover from childhood or, equally repellant, as a moral failure. We want to avoid both invoking irrefutable mental constructs *and* casting moral aspersions at the sufferer, just because that path (psychologism) is wide open to abuse. A physicalist approach, or ontology, seems to be objective, rational, non-judgemental and progressive - you could almost say 'modern'. Who could ask for more? Well, here we run into a problem, as Stoljar's almost forensic dissection concluded:

... there is no version of physicalism that is (a) true and (b) deserves the name... the very considerable influence of physicalism on contemporary philosophy is largely without foundation.

Unfortunately, biological reductionism, the basis of modern biological psychiatry, is very much one of those unfounded versions. Even though it isn't the theme of this book, we will return to this point.

1.2 Dualism, supernatural dualism and its problems. Natural dualism

In contrast to monism, *dualism* states that the universe is of a two-fold nature. The human mind is seen as irreducibly mental in nature, i.e. it has properties which can never be explained by reference to the physical or material universe. Dualism says that, in addition to the material realm of time and space, matter and energy, all governed by the laws of physics (especially the laws of thermodynamics), humans have a mind or mental realm, which is emphatically *not* governed by any physical laws. It has its own laws (we presume there are laws, otherwise the concept of mind is chaotic) which are distinct from those of physics, with no contact at any point: the laws of the physical universe and any mentalist laws constitute separate realms of discourse.

However, because a non-material mind isn't amenable to investigation by the methods and principles of our very successful materialist science, dualism doesn't get a good press. The well-known philosopher, Daniel Dennett (b. 1942), summarised the problem as he saw it:

> My first year in college, I read Descartes' Meditations and was hooked on the mind-body problem. Now here was a mystery. How on earth could my thoughts and feelings fit in the same world with the nerve cells and molecules that made up my brain [7, preface].

Right at the beginning of his education, Dennett concluded they can't. He has spent the rest of his allotted span trying to formulate an alternative, with what would charitably be called limited success. Despite his initial impressions, the fact remains: Yes, we surely have blood and brains and all that physical stuff in our heads but... equally powerful is the belief that there is more to us than mere nerve cells and molecules. We do indeed have "thoughts and feelings," the problem is to give a proper account of them. Philosopher David Oderberg (b. 1963) has long complained not just that dualism is not taken seriously, but that it's actually seen as a joke:

> Dualism... (is) more the object of ridicule than of serious rational engagement. It is held by the vast majority of philosophers to be anything from (and not mutually exclusively) false, mysterious, and bizarre, to obscurantist, unintelligible, and/or dangerous to morals. Its adherents are assumed to be biased, scientifically ill-informed, motivated by prior theological dogma, cursed by metaphysical anachronism, and/or to have taken leave of their senses [8].

Or, as Dennett would say, all of the above. He believes the criticism is justified, and more. Dualism, he says, is crude and infantile magical thinking, the epitome of non-science, a "... hopelessly contradiction-riddled myth..." [7, p 430] that violates the fundamental laws of the universe, creating endless logical problems without solving any:

> Dualism, the idea that a brain cannot be a thinking thing so a thinking thing cannot be a brain ... accepting dualism is giving up... I wiggle my finger by ... what, wiggling my soul?... (mind stuff is) ectoplasm, Wonder Tissue... There is the lurking suspicion that the most attractive feature of mind stuff is its promise of being so mysterious that it keeps science at bay forever ... if dualism is the best we can do, then we can't understand human consciousness [7, p. 37-9].

That more or less sums up Dennett's attitude, but his antagonism is misplaced. The word 'dual' means two-fold. There is nothing in the definition of dualism that implies magic. To paraphrase Richard Watson:

> The crux of dualism is an *apparently unbridgeable gap* between two incommensurable orders of being that must be reconciled if we wish to justify our assumption that the universe is comprehensible [9, emphasis added].

Mind-body dualism says only that there is an apparently unbridgeable gap between the two incommensurable orders of our being, mind and body. The task for any dualist theory is therefore to give a rational account of the apparently immaterial mind *in non-material terms*. That is, it must explain its nature, its origin and how it interacts with the body without relying on physicalist concepts. However, and this is the difficult bit, we have to do so within the modern ontology, meaning without breaching the laws of thermodynamics. That sets an exceedingly high bar. You can understand why people have decided it's easier to abandon dualism: it's just too damned difficult. But to make it worse, I will add a further task: any valid theory of mind must give rise to a formal account of mental disorder. If a theory of mind can't indicate a potential explanation of mental disorder, then it isn't worth pursuing.

There are various types of dualism but the oldest and still the most widespread is *supernatural dualism*. This says that the mind (or soul, or spirit) is not part of the natural, material realm; instead, it belongs to a completely separate, unseen universe with magical properties (magic means forever beyond explanation by natural laws). All religions are based in one form or other of supernatural dualism. For most believers, the most important non-natural property of the mind/soul/spirit is that it will survive the death of the human body. Outright rejection of dualism, such as in Dennett's philippic quoted above, is based on the assumption that all dualism is necessarily supernatural dualism, i.e. that dualism *means* magic, dualism *is* magic. That is, dualism is forever beyond explanation by natural laws and the universe is therefore not comprehensible. Actually, they go a bit further, to argue that dualism is inherently irrational, so accepting dualism means the end of rationalism, where 'rational' equates with 'superior.'

Dennett can afford to pound the table and mock his opponents because, he believes, his stance is superior. Morally superior. Sad to say, he is wrong. Dualism simply means two-fold, and it sets dualists the very difficult task of explaining mind-body interaction, i.e. material-nonmaterial interaction. Of all possible philosophies of mind, it is by far the most difficult. In fact, it is so difficult that it has *bred* physicalism: we live in a monist age *just because* dualism seems forever beyond us. We don't even know where to start with it. So you could liken our "overwhelmingly physicalist or materialist intellectual culture" to the drunk man searching for his lost house key under the street lamp, because that's where the light is. The field of dualism is just all darkness. Fine, say the modernists, let's abandon that field and come over to physicalism, where we have bright lights and sharp tools. This is why people are attracted to monism, not because it has any intrinsic intellectual virtues (c.f. Henry Mencken: "For every complex problem there is an answer that is clear, simple, and wrong").

The alternative to supernatural dualism is known as *natural dualism*. This says that the immaterial mind exists but it is not supernatural and therefore has no magical properties. It arises from the brain by an entirely natural process that we can eventually understand. The emergence of mind from brain is not random or chaotic or mystical, but is entirely rule-governed. Hence, if the brain is damaged or malfunctions in any way, it is perfectly feasible, if not highly likely, that the mind will also be perturbed. Death of an individual's brain will necessarily result in the end of the individual's mind. In any natural dualist theory, as distinct from a supernatural dualist theory, death is final.[2]

1.3 Historical dualism: Descartes, Newton. Watson and behaviorism

Historically, the concept of the mind as a separate entity not governed by the laws of the material realm was brought into sharpest focus by the 17th Century French philosopher and polymath, René Descartes (1596–1650). By a process of systematic doubt, Descartes concluded that the only fact of which he could be absolutely certain was that he existed. He could be deceived or mistaken on any other question but the one point that he could not deny was this: "If I can think, if I can ask 'Do I exist?' then it is indubitable that I do exist." His goal was to use this rock of certainty as the foundation for his entire philosophy.

---

2 As an aside, there is a variant called *mysterianism*, which says that the process by which mind arises from the brain is forever beyond our understanding, we just aren't smart enough. Mysterians set themselves the task of explaining what the mind does without any knowledge of how it does it. Other mysterians see mind as a form of non-reductive physicalism. I don't see how mysterianism can offer a non-reductionist explanation of mental disorder, so we won't bother with it further.

Descartes accepted that the human body is just a bit of fancy clockwork, no different in its nature from the bodies of animals. However, we humans have something else, a mind that controls our bodies with the result that, alone of all animals on earth, we can build, create, speak, write, invent, compose and so on. The mind is a real thing, he said, that can act upon the material world but it is a very strange sort of real thing. It is *res cogitans,* a special "thinking substance" that is…

a   utterly different from material matter;
b   independent of material matter, requiring nothing other than itself to exist;
c   unextended and therefore unlocalised;
d   untouched by and invisible to all physical forces (and therefore unmeasurable); and yet…
e   causally effective.
f   To this, we can add "with an infinite output."

These features are summarised in Table 1.1.

Table 1.1 Summary of properties of Descartes' *res cogitans* or "thinking substance"

Criterion	Descartes
Utterly different from material matter	✓
Exists independently of material matter	✓
Unextended, unlocalised	✓
Invisible to all physical forces	✓
Causally effective	✓
Infinite output	✓
Consistent with laws of thermodynamics	X

One of the major problems in dealing with mind-body interaction is the very rigid definition of science that has come down to us: effectively, "If it can't be measured, it isn't science." Many years ago, a scholar was trying to develop a large-scale theory of how the universe works. In order to complete his model, he needed a force with the following properties:

It is omnipresent, acting across the entire universe;
It is not generated but it inheres in all matter, a brute fact beyond explanation;
It is exceedingly weak but it acts across infinite distances;
It acts upon all matter but is not thereby weakened or dissipated;
It can only be detected by its effect upon matter;
It is always attractive, never repulsive; and…
It cannot be absorbed, transformed, reflected, trapped, stored, evaded or blocked.

At the time, this violated practically all the rules of science, not to mention common sense:

"It is inconceivable," Isaac Newton (1643–1727) complained of his own theory of gravity (1687), "that inanimate Matter should, without the Mediation of something else, which is not material, operate upon, and affect other matter without mutual Contact ... That Gravity should be innate, inherent and essential to Matter, so that one body may act upon another at a distance thro' a Vacuum, without the Mediation of any thing else, by and through which their Action and Force may be conveyed from one to another, is to me so great an Absurdity that I believe no Man who has in philosophical Matters a competent Faculty of thinking can ever fall into it. Gravity must be caused by an Agent acting constantly according to certain laws; but whether this Agent be material or immaterial, I have left to the Consideration of my readers" [10].

For Newton, the concept of action at a distance was the very hallmark of non-science. He was trained in the concepts of science developed by the ancient Greeks, which said that objects moved only if they were either propelled by some inner force or were pushed by an outside force directly touching them, and that the laws governing celestial bodies differed from those governing bodies on earth. Newton threw all this aside. The explosive idea behind his fabled falling apple was not just that the earth attracted and moved the apple *from a distance*, but that the apple also *attracted and moved the earth*. For an educated man of his era, the concept of something the size of the Earth being pulled through empty space was a joke. In fact, it was a very dangerous joke: people were put to death for suggesting that the Church had it wrong.[3] Yet it was a joke that became part of the basis of what we now call modern science. Fifty years earlier, Descartes had wrestled with similar misgivings when he launched his contribution to metaphysics. He was very aware that he had set himself a most difficult task, that of explaining how, if they were so utterly distinct in nature, the two realms (of mind and body) could interact but he had no answer to this. From the beginning, for anybody who wanted to talk about the human mind as a real and effective but peculiar thing, the intractable problem of mind-body interaction seemed a fatal flaw. The constant questioning irked him:

> ...the most ignorant people could, in a quarter of an hour, raise more questions of this kind than the wisest men could deal with in a lifetime; and this is why I have not bothered to answer any of them. These questions presuppose amongst other things an explanation of the union between the soul and the body, which I have not yet dealt with at all (12 January 1646).

Eventually, the problem proved too much and western philosophy drifted away, toward the materialism Descartes probably didn't want. By the latter part of the

---

3 Giordano Bruno (1548–1600) was burned at the stake for suggesting, among other heresies, that the universe is infinite and has no "centre," that stars were far-distant suns that could have planets of their own which, *quele horreur*, could have developed life of their own.

19th century, more and more people were arguing that the mind was either so fundamentally different that it could never be understood by the processes of natural science, or it was just a folk tale, a hangover from a more primitive age. Early in the 20th Century, an American psychologist, John B Watson (1878–1958), announced that it was time for psychology to abandon all hope of understanding the mind, either through analysis or by introspection, as these were just pathways to whimsy. His new science of *behaviorism*, he insisted, will show that observable behaviour is all that counts. The activity of any animal can be fully understood by scientific analysis of observable action, with no reference to unobservables lurking in the darkness between the ears.

By the 1960s, all mentalist psychologies or philosophies were in full-scale retreat, hammered on the one side by the successes of reductionist science and on the other by the very obvious conceptual gap between the physical world and the mental. If we can't see or measure mental life, how can it form the basis of an empirical science? As Oderberg complained, mind-body dualism had become a joke. However, with the concept of a natural dualism, we are trying to duplicate in philosophy of mind Newton's success in physics: to propel what some people see as a joke into the very centre of modern concepts of mind. Needless to say, if it can be done, it would revolutionise our concept of science, quite as much as Newton's theories revolutionised the science of his day.

As a preliminary, we should note two caveats or warnings on Descartes' work by philosopher Gary Hatfield:

> Caveat (1): Those new to the study of Descartes should engage his own works in some detail prior to developing a view of his legacy.

This could almost have been written for certain well-known philosophers who haven't taken to heart Descartes' concept of systematic doubt, at least as it applies to their own work. The second is more general and is really common sense, although often overlooked:

> Caveat (2): In general, it is rare for a philosopher's positions and arguments to remain the same across an entire life.

Philosophers are like everybody else, they have projects which they develop over their lifetimes, the only difference being that their projects are ideas. Naturally, their views change as they mature; naturally, they struggle with difficult concepts and try to refine their work to eliminate errors or inconsistencies; and in this respect, Descartes was no exception. However, he worked under a much greater pressure than simply the intellectual, as he lived in the shadow of the trial of Galileo Galilei (1564–1642) for heresy by the Church in Rome in 1633.

At the time of the trial, Descartes was about to publish a major treatise in three parts, entitled *The World*, but he withdrew it when he realised his arguments in favour of the Copernican model of the universe would be condemned. Two parts of it have survived but, from his writings in his *Discourse on the Method of Science*, there seems little doubt that he knew people could interpret his work as heading toward an unalloyed materialism. This was a major problem to him as he was devout but he was also committed to the idea of letting the work take him where it wanted. As a result, he spent most of the latter part of his life in the Netherlands and other Protestant regions to avoid a collision with the Inquisition.

1.4 Thinking things vs. thinking substance

The essence of material matter, Descartes said, is extension: that it can be seen, measured, weighed, cut in bits and put in bottles flows from that one point. Those were the limits of its properties. A stone can be measured and weighed and broken into bits but it can't do anything else. The essence of the immaterial soul is thought. It could not be measured, weighed or seen but it was nonetheless real in that it could act upon real material objects: I decide to break this stone into bits, and that's what happens. But how can this come to pass? If the thinking stuff has no weight, it can't push on the brain to activate it, even though that was part of Descartes' rather skimpy account. He suggested that the soul acted upon the only midline or non-duplicated structure in the brain, the pineal gland. The mechanics of his scheme aren't relevant here because it was manifestly impossible, as he himself recognised. Immaterial thinking stuff cannot act upon unthinking material stuff just because it can gain no traction on it: imagine a jellyfish trying to move a large boulder. The whole point of a substance is that it has no internal structure; starting from any point within it, the substance is uniform in all directions.

This is the basis of the scorn heaped upon Rene Descartes by modern philosophers. The problem is so blindingly obvious that early in his first semester at college, Freshman Dennett could see it. But I suggest that it did indeed blind him because, had he gone back to the original French edition from 1637, and the Latin translation which appeared soon after, it's clear that something strange happened. In French, Descartes used the term *chose pensante* more or less interchangeably with the expression *substance pensante*. The same thing happens in the Latin version, translated by Etienne de Courcelles, a French Protestant minister and translator (I don't know why Descartes didn't translate his own work as he was fluent in Latin and classical Greek from an early age, but perhaps he had better things to do). Here, we find *substantia cogitans*, thinking substance, and *res cogitans* or thinking thing. However, as it comes down to us in English, we find only *thinking substance*. There is no sign of the *thinking thing,* wherein lies the problem because, by definition, an immaterial substance can't act upon a material substance. A thinking substance is *sui generis*, ontologically sufficient unto itself, meaning it does not depend on anything else to exist. By definition, it is apart from the material world: if it were not, it wouldn't be immaterial.

If we accept the English translation, then it would seem Descartes' project was doomed. There is no conceivable way for immaterial substances to act upon the physical world, just because the closed nature of the physical world excludes them from having any effect. Its laws don't leave any loopholes, the door is slammed shut, as Descartes himself appeared to understand. If, on the other hand, we define an immaterial *thinking thing* as something that, by an as yet unspecified means, can act upon the physical world, then perhaps the door is left, if not wide open, then just slightly ajar. Intuitively, a "thing" has an internal structure, it is composed of parts or other, smaller things. That is, if there is some element involved in the construction of the thinking thing that has some form of commonality with the physical universe, then there may be a path from the one to the other. Of course, there remains the old problem of keeping the leprechauns out, but we'll come back to this point.

Can there be a model of an immaterial thinking thing or entity that is causally efficacious on the material world? Conceivably, there can be and, I will argue, there certainly is. It doesn't require any metaphysical gymnastics to show how it acts on the body because we have been using the concepts for a very long time. In fact, it is so obvious that we have overlooked it. However, in order to see that, we have to take a fairly long detour through some rather arcane matters, but we will not lose sight of the central point of this book, the idea of the mind as a real, effective but immaterial thing generated by that most amazing organ, the human brain.

References

[1] Kupfer DJ, Kuhl EA, Wuisin L (2013). Psychiatry's integration with medicine: the role of DSM5. *Annual Review of Medicine* 64: 385–392.

[2] Insel TR, Cuthbert BN, Garvey M, et al (2010). Research Domain Criteria (RDoC): toward a new classification framework for research on mental disorders. Commentary. *American Journal of Psychiatry*, 167: 748–751.

[3] McHugh PR, Slavney PR (1998). *The Perspectives of Psychiatry*. Baltimore: Johns Hopkins U Press.

[4] McLaren N (2013). Psychiatry as Ideology. *Ethical Human Psychology and Psychiatry* 15: 7–18.

[5] Harrington A (2020). *Mind Fixers: Psychiatry's Troubled Search for the Biology of Mental Illness*. New York: Norton.

[6] Stoljar D (2010). *Physicalism*. Oxford: Routledge.

[7] Dennett DC (1991). *Consciousness Explained*. London: Penguin Books.

[8] Oderberg DS (2005). Hylemorphic Dualism, in Paul EF, Miller FD, Paul J: *Personal Identity*. Cambridge: University Press.

[9] Watson RA (1995), p210 in Audi R (Ed.) *The Cambridge Dictionary of Philosophy*. Cambridge: University Press.

[10] Newton I (1687). *Letters to Bentley, 1692/3*. Quoted in Maxwell JC (1876). On Action At A Distance, in *Scientific Papers of James Clerk Maxwell*, vol 2, LIV, p. 311. *Proceedings of the Royal Institution of Great Britain*, Vol VII. http://www.informationphilosopher.com/solutions/scientists/maxwell/action_at_a_distance.html

2   Toward a natural dualism

A new scientific truth does not triumph by convincing its opponents and making them see the light, but rather because its opponents eventually die, and a new generation grows up that is familiar with it.

Max Planck (1858–1947)
The philosophy of physics (1936)

I don't pretend we have all the answers. But the questions are certainly worth thinking about.

Arthur C Clarke (1917–2008)

2.1 The problem with reductionism

The primary claim of reductionist biological psychiatry is that a full knowledge of the brain, as revealed by the concepts and technology of ordinary laboratory science, will tell us all we need to know about mental disorder, leaving no significant questions unanswered. Look at this "postition statement" from a major undergraduate text on neurosciences:

> In neuroscience, there is no need to separate *mind* from *brain*; once we fully understand the individual and concerted actions of brain cells, we will understand our mental abilities [1, p. 24].

For a number of reasons, this is a bold stance to take. First, questions on the nature of mind are metaphysical, meaning they are not the sorts of questions that empirical or ordinary laboratory science can answer. Anybody who claims that physical sciences can explain all possible questions is making a major metaphysical claim, which has to be justified, not treated as *fait accompli*. Second, nobody knows what it means to say the mind is a physical thing. Third, nobody has ever offered any suggestion of how this program might be implemented. Four, if we apply this to that familiar object, the digital computer, it implies there is no such thing as software, which would probably be news to some very wealthy people. Finally, the historical evidence is that the search for the physical causes of mental

DOI: 10.4324/9781003183792-2

disorder is just a breathtakingly expensive, high-tech search for the end of a rainbow. As soon as somebody makes an advance in basic molecular biology, psychiatrists pounce on it and try to apply it to their field. In the main, they don't understand what they are doing and the results are uniformly dismal, but that never deters anybody in the industry.

It is beyond doubt that there is something in us that doesn't fit in the physical world: I look outside my window at the clear blue sky, and I see *something*, but there isn't a speck of blue inside my head. The only problem is to give an account of it; it has to be explained, not dismissed. The earliest concept of rational or non-spiritual dualism, Descartes's substance dualism, invoked two inherently different substances, the material and the thinking, each of which required nothing other than itself to exist. This immediately ran into the problem of how these would interact, a problem which, *pace* Dennett and so many others, Descartes himself recognised from the outset. However, if we go back to the original French and Latin versions of his work, we find that he wasn't wedded to the dual *substance* model as the English translations imply. The mind is *res cogitans,* a thinking *thing* made of a substance whose only known property is thought, although that gives no clues as to how it might interact with the material world.

In order to solve this ancient dilemma, we need to find a commonality, an element or feature common to both realms, the material and the immaterial, to serve as a bridge or point of contact by which communication can take place. And, of course, phrasing it that way directs our search to a model that wasn't available to Descartes in 1640, or in 1840, or even 1940, but is now commonplace. It's our good fortune that the first formal theoretical account of the common element between the physical body and the thinking "thing" was published in 1948, and it has since grown into something very, very big. The idea was always there, of course, but it is like the nose on our faces: we all depend utterly upon it, yet it is so blindingly obvious that we don't see it. Giving a proper account of the bridge between mind and body will require a further historical detour.

2.2 Boole and dual-valued calculus

In 1847, a young, largely self-taught and largely unknown English mathematician working in the remote town of Cork, in the far south of Ireland, published a small pamphlet titled *A Mathematical Analysis of Logic.* At the age of just 32yrs, George Boole (1815–64) outlined the revolutionary notion of translating logic into a mathematical form. At the time, logic was seen as an intellectual discipline based in rules formulated by the classic Greek philosophers. There was no order to their schema, and the rules didn't fit into a larger structure, so applying them left plenty of scope for imagination – and dispute. Boole wanted to show that reasoning (the process of using logical methods to reach valid conclusions) is non-metaphysical in nature and, as an independent and universal science, could therefore be reframed in a mathematical notation that anybody could learn and apply. Boole wasn't happy with this little introduction and, over the next seven years, expanded the project greatly in a provocatively-titled book, *An Investigation of the Laws of Thought* (1854), [2].

His concerns were general. He started with the idea that humans can reason, meaning infer valid conclusions from limited evidence. Valid inference, or what we would now call logic itself, was, he believed, neither random nor a mystical process that only the cognoscenti could understand, but could be formalised into a series of laws. Critically, he argued that these were independent of the nature of mind itself. Therefore, he explicitly avoided relying on what he called metaphysical presumptions of mind, and actually says nothing about it. He was concerned with how the mind does its job, not so much with what it is.

170 years later, Boole's book is still prodigiously difficult to read, not least because it requires considerable familiarity with logic and algebra, but also because it is written in that turgid and frequently opaque style which marked the era.[1] It is also difficult because he seems to have intuitively grasped the notion of a mathematised logic early, and then spent most of the remainder of his short life trying to cast it in the form of a mathematical proof. Thus, it isn't easy to see how he reached some of his conclusions. Perhaps he wasn't sure of his proofs himself, he just knew they were right. His widow said of him:

> My husband told me that when he was a lad of seventeen a thought struck him suddenly, which became the foundation of all his future discoveries. It was a flash of psychological insight into the conditions under which a mind most readily accumulates knowledge...
>
> George afterwards learned, to his great joy, that the same conception of the basis of Logic was held by Leibnitz, the contemporary of Newton.... nearly all the logicians and mathematicians ignored the statement that the book was meant to throw light on the nature of the human mind; and treated the formula entirely as a wonderful new method of reducing to logical order masses of evidence about external fact.

By his astounding intellectual achievement, Boole showed that logic could be rewritten in a mathematical form to become a formal process involving no interpretation and no intuition. Logic was no longer an art form but followed a rule-governed and stepwise progress that did not allow any deviation, or what we would now call an *algorithm*. The point of an algorithm is that, by following the instructions, intelligence and creativity are trumped by blind obedience. Unfortunately, Boole died of pleurisy a few years later, in 1864, aged just forty-nine, but the impact of his thirty-two years of productive work has been incalculable. It took a while for his discoveries to be fully understood and

---

1 For example, he freely used the rhetorical device called litotes, affirming something in understatement by denying its opposite; *and* he does it not infrequently in interposed subordinate clauses.

appreciated, but he was one of the outstanding figures in that century whose work has changed the world.

Boole's "science of logic" was based on the notion of a *dual-valued calculus*, originally developed by Gottfried Leibniz (1646–1716). A calculus is defined as *any formal system in which symbolic expressions are manipulated according to fixed rules*. The word comes from the Latin word *calculus*, or stone, as the first such systems were simply piles of stones used by traders in the market, e.g. five small stones equals one big one. In Boole's logical calculus, there were only two values: all, or nothing. He wrote these as 1 and 0 but it must be understood that 1 is not the *number* one, it is shorthand for "all, the universe of objects." He could equally have used A for all, or U for universe. By applying another set of values, of true and false, the theorems that flowed from his dual-valued calculus formed the basis of modern propositional logic. The operations of a dual-valued calculus with the values T (for true) and F (false) are known as *logical operations*. The input of a logical operation consists of one or more propositions while the output is also a proposition.

So what are his "Laws of Thought"? They just are the laws governing a dual-valued calculus, most of which he derived and proved himself. Insofar as human thought can undertake any process of reasoning, he claimed, it must rely *in some sense* on the fundamental logical rules that he described. That is, his laws of logic, as he understood them, were also the laws of reasoning, or thought. We would now be a little more circumspect, but even if the human mind doesn't function using just his laws, the rules of his dual-valued calculus adequately summarise the operations of human reasoning. Different method, perhaps, but since reasoning is universal, same outcome. As long as they reach the same conclusions, the distinction between the two systems would be a distinction without a difference.

2.3 Truth tables and logical operators

At about the same time, in England, another mathematician, Charles Babbage (1791–1871), developed the concept of a machine that could perform arithmetic calculations. Working with Countess Ada Lovelace (1815–1852), Byron's only legitimate child, who is sometimes called the first computer programmer, Babbage formulated the principles of mechanical computation. While he showed that a calculating machine was feasible, his plans were never fully realised during his life time. This took the processes of reasoning further down the track of mechanisation. In the era of Darwin's *Origin of Species*, humans were losing their aura of mysticism.

In the early part of the 20th Century, logicians formalised the idea of *truth tables*. This is a matrix showing how the outcome (truth value) of a logical operation (i.e. the operations of a dual-valued calculus with the values T and F) varies according to the truth or falsity of its inputs. Although Boole certainly had an implicit idea of the concept, the earliest example of a truth matrix is thought to be in the private papers of the American logician, Charles Peirce (1839–1914), from about 1887. A lot of the early work on truth values was done by the logician and philosopher, Gottlob Frege (1848–1925). Truth tables themselves were expanded by the German philosopher, Ludwig Wittgenstein (1889–1951), although others, including Bertrand Russell (1872–1970), worked on them at about the same time.

For each logical operation, a table can be compiled that shows how its output varies with the truth status of each of its inputs. Since most logical operators work on two inputs or propositions, they are known as binary operators. The only *unary operator* is *negation*, which acts on a single input proposition and simply inverts its truth value. Thus, if the input proposition is true, e.g. *Ice is cold*, then clearly its negation, i.e. the assertion *Ice is not cold*, is false.

All other logical operators are *binary*, meaning they work on two propositions, as in:

P1: Ice is cold.
P2: The sun is hot.

We can combine these sentences via the binary operator known as conjunction to give:

Ice is cold *and* the sun is hot;
P1 ∧ P2 (there are different notations but this is the most common).

Because each of the inputs is true, the conjoined sentence is true, written as:

T: P1 ∧ P2

We now want to know what happens to the combined sentence if one of its components is false, as in:

Ice is cold *and* the sun is not hot.

That is, if one element of the sentence is false, what happens to the truth value of the *whole* sentence? Clearly, in this case, the whole sentence is false. This is a simple example but mostly, truth isn't quite so easily determined. For all possible combinations of truth and falsity for the conjunction of two propositions, A and B, the truth table or matrix is shown in Table 2.1.

Table 2.1 Truth Table for Conjunction

A	B	A ∧ B
T	T	T
T	F	F
F	T	F
F	F	F

The compound sentence is true only in the specific case that both its elements are true. For any other input, the whole sentence is rendered false.

Another very important operator is logical implication, the conditional *If A, then B* (e.g. If the bulbs are flowering, then it's spring). The abbreviated version is A → B. In common language, this is usually taken to mean that if A is true, B is causally true but, in logic, it can be just association. It simply means "If A is true, then B is also true." The proposition A → B is false only in the case where B is false. All other combinations are logically true, even if the assertion doesn't make sense, as in Table 2.2.

Table 2.2 Truth Table for Logical Implication

A	B	A → B
T	T	T
T	F	F
F	T	T
F	F	T

Truth tables have been constructed for all of the sixteen possible logical operators relating two autonomous propositions. Truth functions can be combined to duplicate the outcome of the primary operators, e.g. (A → B) is logically equivalent to ¬(A ∧ ¬B) and to (¬A ∨ B) (where ¬ = *not*, and ∨ = *or*). This point directly refutes the claim that the output of a computation is strictly related to or reducible to its physical substrate. Computations can be instantiated by many different means, perhaps even infinite, so there cannot be a necessary reductionist relationship between the propositions and their implementation. On this point, universal reductionism fails.

The truth table for the disjunctive operator (or = ∨) is not entirely intuitive. In common language, there are two ways of using "or," as follow:

a. You can have tea or coffee (meaning You can have tea, or you can have coffee, or you can have both if you want to be a pest).
b. Smith is dead or alive (but he can't be both).

The first use is called 'inclusive or' while the second is 'exclusive or.' In common language, we tend to distinguish these two uses of 'or' by saying "For your holiday, you can either go to Rome or you can go to Patagonia," the implication being you can't do both. However, in logic, if we try to restrict the disjunctive operator to exclusive or (as in 'Either one or the other but not both'), we run into all sorts of complexities. Thus, the word 'or' in logic is inclusive, meaning "*either* A *or* B *or both*." The disjunctive operator 'or' does *not* exclude conjunction. It is therefore *logically* possible that Smith can indeed be both dead *and* alive at the same time. However, bear in mind that the set of people who are both dead *and* alive is empty. It is conceptually feasible but, like pink elephants, it just happens to be that there aren't any.

Truth tables are important for two reasons. In the first place, they again show that the processes of logic are essentially very ordinary mechanical steps with no room for imagination. Schoolboys can learn them, so logic is no longer the exclusive domain of Olympian intellects - and the egos that often go with them. The second point is that the laws governing truth functors are not *physical* laws. Logic exists in a semantic world, or world of meaning, entirely separate from the material realm of physics, thermodynamics etc. Most importantly, this does not mean "anything goes," as the world of meaning is governed by the laws of semantics of its particular system: "It has its own laws which are distinct from those of physics, with no cross-over at any point." Semantic laws cannot be reduced to physical laws. These points are critically important in arriving at a natural dualist theory of mind.

2.4 Turing's universal computer

Moving on, in 1936, a young British mathematician, Alan Turing (1912–1954), published a paper in which he outlined the essential principles of machine-based intelligence. A few pages into a forbiddingly complex paper, he stated:

> It is possible to invent a single machine which can be used to compute any computable sequence [3].

He expanded on his concepts in a further paper, in 1950, in which he asked "Can machines think?" His answer was, essentially, it doesn't matter. If they can fool us, that's good enough. But how could a machine fool humans into believing that it could think? Turing's startlingly simple answer forms the basis of modern computing. Any question that a human can ask, he said, can be broken down into a series of sub-questions. These can be further broken down, again and again, until all that is left is a series of questions that are so elementary that a dumb machine can answer them simply by, for example, choosing which is the larger of two numbers. It is wholly a matter of mechanics, not of intellect.

The idealised machine he proposed consisted of just four parts, an input-output tape, a read-write head, a memory store, and an executive or control unit. The tape is divided into squares, or cells, that hold only one of two tokens, either 0 or 1, Yes or No, On or Off, etc. That is, his machine operated in a dual-valued calculus. The machine's read-write head can perform only four operations: erase, write, move forward, move back. As the tape clicks forward, the mechanism scans what is written in each cell and conveys this to the executive unit which checks the memory and decides what to do. It can either leave the token as it is, or erase it and write the other, but it cannot do anything else. The machine then clicks to the next cell.

The simplest version of the machine would have a fixed memory, or what we would now call 'hard-wired.' It could only perform one function so if anybody wanted it to work on another task, the memory would have to be physically taken apart and rebuilt. Turing reasoned that if a machine could be given enough memory, and its instructions or program were themselves written on the input tape, then it would be able to calculate any known mathematical problem (although we may not live long enough to know it). This he called a 'universal computing machine' although we now know it as a Turing machine.

The real value of its ability to calculate mathematical problems was that, following from Boole's discoveries, all questions that can be answered by a process of logic could now be answered by a machine implementing an algorithm. Any questions humans can ask, even questions of morality or value, can be rephrased in logical form, so a machine can answer any question a human can ask. That is, in terms of thinking, machines can potentially do as well as humans, and certainly much faster and more accurately.

Turing understood that a machine's output could be fed back to modify its process; he saw that the output of one machine could become the input of the next; and that the output of one machine could reprogram the next machine. Thus, his finite machines could potentially generate an infinite output. At that stage, of course, there was no mechanism of putting his concept into practice but, just a few years later, using the principles he had outlined, he and his group built the first electronic computer (known as Colossus). By 1950, he was able to state:

> I believe that at the end of the century, the use of words and general educated opinion will have altered so much that one will be able to speak of machines thinking without expecting to be contradicted [4].

In fact, it was much sooner than that.

What is the relevance of all this mathematical talk in answering the question of whether biology or psychology causes mental disorder? The answer lies in an apparently cryptic remark from the psychologist Philip Johnson-Laird (b. 1936):

> Any scientific theory of the mind has to treat it as an automaton (1983).

This means that if we wish to give a scientific account of the mind, we have to be able to explain mental activity in mechanical (non-mental) terms, otherwise we simply set up a circular pseudo-explanation. For example, people sometimes try to explain vision as an internal TV screen watched by a little person sitting inside the head who decides what to do. But this explains nothing, it only shifts whatever requires to be explained deeper inside the head. We now have to explain how the little person sees: another little man inside his head? Remember the couplet about dog fleas:

> Dog fleas have little fleas, upon their backs to bite 'em.
> And the little fleas have littler fleas, and so *ad infinitum*.

This sort of 'explanation,' where the point to be explained just keeps receding further and further away, is known as an infinite regress. An infinite regress may look scientific but it has no explanatory value, so it is never valid. So if we want to explain human decision-making, we need to make sure we never take the first step on the slippery slope to an infinite regress. This is the real problem with dualism, not that it is necessarily magic but that it can lead to an infinite regress.

To finish this section, recall that any dualist theory starts off with a major handicap, that some very influential people think dualism is a joke. Just like Kupfer, Insel, Dennett and so many others, the mind of a biological reductionist is already made up. He doesn't want anybody telling him that his narrow, reductionist idea of science will never deliver the goods. So, in proposing a natural dualist theory for psychiatry, we need to outline in the most tedious detail every step from start to finish, to show that there is no place for magic. Dennett actually makes this point himself in a cartoon on p38 of his book, *Consciousness Explained* [5]. A physicist has written a long formula on the board. In the middle is a section that says 'Then a miracle occurs.' A colleague points to this section and says: "I think you should be more explicit at this point." The point is crucial: if we want to give a natural dualist account of mind, we have to show that human mentality arises from insentient neurons blindly doing their thing without relying on mental concepts (begging the question), on miracles (magic) to complete the causal chain, or evading the question by infinite regression. And that, of course, is the definition of complexity: Individually simple agents produce a complex output without central control.

2.5 Shannon and logic gates

Meanwhile, over at the University of Michigan, an even younger graduate student had just submitted a thesis that has been called "the most important masters thesis in history." Like other keen young engineers in 1937, twenty-one year old Claude Shannon (1916–2001) was interested in the most complex engineering issue of the day, telephony. The big question was how to organise the switches in the large telephone exchanges that were being built as phone lines snaked across the continent. Shannon was an unusual student, and not just because of his prodigious intellect. He was quite a distant person and had a number of odd habits, including riding a monocycle around his university. Another unusual point was that he had just completed a double major in mathematics and engineering. As part of his maths course, he had attended lectures on logic, so he was familiar with recent developments.

Two engineering problems in particular exercised him: firstly, how to make sure that a system of switches was the most economical of all possibilities, and second, how to write a formula for a switch to do a specific job. Shannon's solution to these problems was remarkable but, while he was writing it, he outlined a profoundly important point: that certain combinations of switches reproduced the input-output ratios of the major truth tables. For example, the input-output pattern of an inverter switch was exactly the same as for the truth table of the logical operation of negation. Very quickly, he wrote the formulae for a range of switches using the two values of *On* and *Off*. This showed a precise, one-to-one relationship with the operations of logic:

Table 2.3 "Analogue between the calculus of propositions and the symbolic relay analysis." Adapted from Shannon, CE (1937) [6]

Symbol	Interpretation in relay circuits	Interpretation in the Calculus of Propositions
X	The circuit X	The proposition X
0	The circuit is closed	The proposition is false
1	The circuit is open	The proposition is true
X+Y	The series connection of circuits X and Y	The proposition which is true if either X or Y is true
XY	The parallel connection of circuits X and Y	The proposition which is true if both X and Y are true
X'	The circuit which is open when X is closed, and closed when X is open	The contradictory of proposition X
=	The circuits open and close simultaneously	Each proposition implies the other.

Two important notes to this table. First, a semantic quibble: In his title to this table, he used the term 'analogue.' In fact, it is a homologue, as he immediately acknowledged when he referred to it as "a perfect analogy."

> ....it is evident that a *perfect analogy* exists between the calculus of switching circuits and ... symbolic logic. ... Any expression formed with the operations of addition, multiplication, and negation represents explicitly a circuit containing only series and parallel connections ... Any circuit is represented by a set of equations, the terms of the equations representing the various switches and relays of the circuit. ... It is also possible to use the analogy between Boolean algebra and relay circuits in the opposite direction, *i.e., to represent logical relations by means of electric circuits* (emphasis added).

Second, be aware that in talking about switches being open or closed, the flow of current is the opposite of what we would expect. For example, when a gate is open, the sheep can run through it. When a tap is open, water flows. When a window is open, air flows. When a politician's mouth is open, nonsense flows. But when an electric switch is open, i.e. the input and output leads are not in contact, then current *doesn't* flow.

Bearing that in mind, look again at the quote above. Shannon's last sentence is critical. In practical terms, his astounding insight meant he could build circuits to perform logical operations according to Boole's *Laws of Thought*. His arrays of switches were in fact little logic devices or, because he used a dual-valued logic, Boolean switches. We now call them logic gates and they are the basis of computing as we know it. Thus, Shannon theoretically justified the mechanism that Turing had needed. The *and* gate had actually been devised in 1924, while Turing and his group in the UK discovered them independently (see the fascinating biography of Turing by Andrew Hodges [7]). Shannon's work mechanised Boole's calculus of logical operations generally, which is exactly what Boole and, later, Babbage had intended.

During World War Two, Shannon was fully occupied working on the complexities of anti-aircraft fire control mechanisms. Meanwhile, in Britain, Turing was the major force in decoding the German Enigma codes. They actually met in 1943 when Turing visited the US but it seems unlikely they were able to discuss their work in any detail. It was not until after the War that Shannon returned to the theoretical concepts behind machine-based logic. In 1948, he published a major paper in which he outlined the mathematical basis for communication, or what is now (incorrectly) known as the theory of information. Right at the beginning, he specified his interest as a question of the mechanism by which two entities can exchange information:

> The fundamental problem of communication is that of reproducing at one point either exactly or approximately a message selected at another point. Frequently the messages have meaning; that is they refer to or are correlated according to some system with certain physical or conceptual entities. These semantic aspects of communication are irrelevant to the engineering problem [8].

As a communications engineer rather than a semanticist, Shannon's concern lay in squirting signals down a wire in such a way as to be sure that what came out the other end was exactly what had gone in. As he said, he had no direct interest in the meaning of what went in. Engineers are like that: to a hydraulics engineer, it matters not whether what goes through his pipe is wine or sewage, the practical problems are the same. This point becomes of critical importance in a theory of language.

We can now see how, by a series of discoveries, building upon each other over a period of a hundred years, the hitherto mystical but quintessentially human process of reasoning was reduced to the blind operations of dumb mechanism. Very quickly, people understood that when it came to logic, anything a human could do, a machine could do, and probably better. It would seem, then, that this is the very essence of reductionism, that dualism must fail because a higher-order process is reduced to a lower-order mechanism. However, that conclusion points to the grievous error at the core of attempts to reduce human mentality to its biological substrate, the brain: the conflation of a process and its underlying mechanism. A process is never a mechanism, and vice versa. They represent different ontological orders, one semantic and the other of thermodynamic organisation. A mechanism is a physical structure which acquits a process, the energy flow goes one way. We cannot reverse a process to produce a mechanism, that's not how the material universe works.

It would appear, then, that the actual process of logic is irreducible. Reductionists still cannot escape Watson's dilemma:

The crux of dualism is an *apparently unbridgeable gap* between two incommensurable orders of being that must be reconciled if we wish to justify our assumption that the universe is comprehensible.

2.6 Causation

We need to look more closely at the notion of incommensurable orders of being, and the easiest way to do this is via the concept of causation. We say event A causes event B when A is both necessary and sufficient for B. That is, B can't occur until A occurs (A is necessary), and if A occurs, nothing else is required for B to occur so it must happen (A is sufficient). We can have simple physical causation, like billiard ball A colliding with another ball B. By its impact, the kinetic energy in the moving ball A is transferred to stationary ball B, causing it to move. Under normal conditions, B won't move unless and until A hits it, then it's impossible for B not to move. This is the standard linear or Newtonian model of mechanics that governs most of our daily lives. By increasing the complexity of the mechanism, we quickly arrive at the vastly complex machines in daily use, up to and including nuclear power stations.

On a similar causative level, we can mix an acid and a carbonate to produce a salt plus water plus carbon dioxide. There is nothing mysterious about this, we understand all the matter and energy inputs that lead to just this outcome. The same applies to biological processes, such as photosynthesis or cardiac contraction. There is nothing magical involved in these events, they require no *élan vital* to complete the causative sequence. Given the particular molecular mechanisms and the energies involved, the events will occur and, all things being equal, can't be stopped. As questions of causation, billiard balls, leaves and hearts are of the same order of being, the material order. Given the physical structure, we can fully explain each event in terms of matter-energy balances in the time-space matrix, relying on no miracles and with no questions remaining.

Fifty million years before the earliest proto-human took its first unsteady steps across the lush plains of East Africa, there were, we are quite sure, winds blowing, rocks banging into each other, waves breaking and leaves on plants growing and dying. At the time, there was absolutely no question of mentality involved in any of these events. A full understanding of the matter-energy elements involved in these physical events and the laws governing them tells us all there is to know about the event. That remains true today, for rocks, trees and sea-slugs. It is also true of machines such as electric locks on doors: pressing the button sends a current through a circuit which closes a switch, triggers an electromagnet or servomotor, and the door swings open. No magic involved. We understand the mechanics of heavier-than-air flight, of antibiotics and immunisation, conception and contraception, birth and death. Again, no miracles are needed to explain the chain of causation.

Now let's go to the village of Spiennes, in south-west Belgium. Scattered over an area of about 100ha are millions of fragments of flint which do not come from surface deposits but which were mined in shafts up to 10m deep and brought to the surface. Four thousand years ago, these mines were the major source of flint knives, axe heads and arrow tips for the Neolithic people of the region. Today, we can give a precise description of the energy expended in shaping a piece of flint, the muscles involved as the craftsman seizes a piece of rock, the exact biochemical pathways by which his muscles contract, how the fracture lines spread through the cryptocrystalline structure of the stone, on and on. All of this we know in great detail as examples of events causally governed by the laws of the physical universe. The only element missing in the chain of explanation is … Why?

Why did the workers go to such great efforts, not to mention the terrible risks, to bring the lumps of flint to the surface? Why did they strike the stones at just this angle, to produce just this edge, then shape it again and again until it yielded an edge that would cut wood or sinews? This is the human element that cannot be explained by the laws of the physical universe, the human explanatory element that distinguishes us from rocks, trees and sea-slugs. Rocks tumbling down a hillside don't need a *Why*, just as wintry gusts have no *Wherefore*. The interaction of the DNA of a seed with its environment gives a full account of the *Why* of trees; while sea-slugs are only a few degrees more complex than mosses and represent no conceptual problems. However, the DNA of *Homo sapiens* does not give any account of making flint axes, or wedding cakes, nor of the concept of monotheism or of the "Analogue between the calculus of propositions and the symbolic relay analysis." Nor is this information coded at a submolecular level: atoms do not have a sense of humour.

The explanation of the flints being brought to ground level is just this: "Because the miners wanted to." That's all, but this construct does not derive or flow from our physical structure, it requires some further explanation. This is not a case of "explaining each event in terms of matter-energy balances in the time-space matrix, with no questions remaining." Looking at all the flint fragments on the ground raises questions which the laws of physics can never explain, just because they don't apply. That is, as soon as we use mental concepts such as "wanted to" to complete an explanatory sequence, we have all the evidence we need of "two incommensurable orders of being." Our task now is to attempt to reconcile them.

My proposal is that the path set out by the work of Boole, of Turing and of Shannon, leads to a dualist model that escapes the Scylla of incompatible substances on the one hand, and the Charybdis of an infinite regress on the other. The model is built around the concept of information, a real thing that can be apprehended, stored, processed and transmitted to act upon the real world, yet which is also immaterial and unextended. Some people, however, have trouble with this notion, and part of the difficulty is that information is so much *part of us* that we take it for granted. We can't conceive of ourselves stripped of our informational capacity, therefore we don't see how pervasive and effective it is, how it shapes our perception of the universe. For example, look at the old question: a rock falls down a cliff in a distant desert where there are no living creatures of any kind, and is smashed to pieces. Does it cause a sound? Similarly, does gold have the property of being yellow?

In each case, the answer is no. The impact of the rock certainly produces a sudden pattern of pressure changes in the air but unless there is a suitably-equipped entity to perceive and process those changes, then there is no experience called "sound." Sound is not a thing "out there," it is wholly an event "in here." To us, sound is so much part of the universe as we experience and understand it that we struggle to imagine a world without it. Similarly, pure gold reflects light at a wavelength of about 585nm (~515THz). However, that light has no colour until it strikes a particular sort of receptor and the ensuing volley of digital impulses is processed by a suitably-equipped data processor. Colour exists in a mental space, not in physical space. What colour is ultraviolet? No colour. The energy of a particular part of the electromagnetic spectrum isn't colour until information about it gets into a mind, and a mind is not a brain (the properties of a mind are not those of a brain, and vice versa). The *intentions* to produce a flint knife, or ring a bell, or write a poem on yellow daffodils, are not properties of the material world, even though all intentions arise through, and are effected, *just because* of that world.

2.7 An informational realm

The informational realm must not be taken for granted. Arrays of switches functioning as Boolean logic gates don't know what they're doing. Switches are insensate; they simply take packets of impulses and send them in different directions according to their settings. If the settings are such that the impulses simply go round and round in infinite circles, or flick on and off randomly, nothing but heat and noise will emerge from the switches. However, the same switches can also be realigned so that their input/output ratios mimic what we call the processes of logic in a dual-valued calculus.

In just that case, what then emerges is not heat and noise but is a highly specific and, above all, novel output, one which is both about the world and (given a suitable three pin plug) able to act on it. Such outputs are otherwise known as information. That is, letting the switches function randomly achieves nothing. However, by using different settings so that the packets of impulses are manipulated according to predetermined rules, or calculus, the switches can solve major problems of logic *with no further energy input*. That is, once a switching device is active, it can either contribute to the slow winding-down of the universe with no measurable change, or it can increase knowledge, but it does this *without* breaching the laws of thermodynamics. The logical function "hitches a ride" on the physical switch without using any extra energy.

> *Thus, semantic operations can be performed at no additional cost to the matter-energy balance of the universe. It is by this means that the essential duality of the universe comes into being. Until this point, there is only one set of laws for the universe. Immediately thereafter, and with no change of entropy, there are two ontologically distinct sets, the physical laws and the semantic laws.*

Human knowledge is the original free lunch, but the universe is not of a dual nature unless and until these specific switching devices are in action. To rephrase that, suitably-organised Boolean-type switches are both necessary and sufficient to generate semantic properties in the world as we know it (there may be other universes where this isn't true but we're not talking about them). When those properties occur in a human, we call them mental properties. It follows that this novel dual element of the universe can flicker in and out of existence as the switches are turned on, off, and on again.

If the settings of the switch array can be varied according to its informational input, then Turing's concept of the "universal computing machine" is realised. Again, this is achieved wholly within the constraints of the laws of thermodynamics. Given suitable switching devices, information can be manipulated without changing the matter-energy status of the devices themselves. Switches consume energy; what they achieve with that energy is "irrelevant to the engineering problem," to paraphrase Shannon. A switching device could write a sonnet, design a nuclear bomb or just generate white noise at the same matter-energy cost, it's all the same to the dumb switches. Switches don't "know" anything: they are the elements of Johnson-Laird's automata.

Thus generated, the dual nature of the universe is both necessary and sufficient to explain the "Why?" of human actions. A purely physicalist explanation of human behaviour is never complete. There is always a further element that can only be explained by the informational content of the semantic space generated by the high-speed switching of data, a content that accounts for intention, meaning, symbolism and significance. An appeal to a dualist element to complete the chain of causation is not "magical thinking." Indeed, the only justification for appealing to physicalist explanations is to appear "less magical than thou," of which Dennett's oft-repeated anti-dualist tirades are a case in point.

References

[1] Bear M, Connors B, Paradiso M (2016). *Neuroscience: Exploring the Brain*. 4th Edition. Burlington, MA: Jones & Bartlett.

[2] Boole G (1854) *An Investigation of the Laws of Thought, on which are Founded the Mathematical Theories of Logic and Probabilities*. Dover Classics of Science and Mathematics. New York: Dover. Also available through Google Books.

[3] Turing AM (1937). On computable numbers, with an application to the Entscheidungsproblem. *Proceedings of the London Mathematical Society (1936– 37) Series* 2; 42:230–265 (now available on line; see author entry in Wikipedia).

[4] Turing AM (1950). Computing machinery and intelligence. *Mind*; 59: 433–460.

[5] Dennett DC (1991). *Consciousness Explained*. London: Penguin Books (1993).

[6] Shannon CE (1937). *A Symbolic Analysis of Relay and Switching Circuits*, unpublished MS Thesis, Massachusetts Institute of Technology, Aug. 10, 1937. Available at: http://dspace.mit.edu/bitstream/handle/1721.1/11173/34541425.pdf?sequence=1 Accessed June 24th 2012.

[7] Hodges A (1983) *Alan Turing: The enigma*. London: Vintage Press.

[8] Shannon CE (1948) A Mathematical Theory of Communication. *Bell System Technical Journal* 27: 379–423, 623–656 (July, October).

3 The mind as an informational space

How it is that anything so remarkable as a state of consciousness comes about as a result of irritating nervous tissue, is just as unaccountable as the appearance of the Djinn when Aladdin rubbed his lamp.

Thomas Huxley (1825–1925)
The Elements of Physiology 1869

Nature in her unfathomable designs has mixed us of clay and flame, of brain and mind, that the two things hang indubitably together and determine each other's being, but how or why, no mortal may ever know.

William James (1842–1910)
Principles of Psychology, Ch. VI

3.1 Defining informational space

Thus far, we have established a case for there being two distinct realms of reality in the universe. The first is the everyday realm of matter-energy interactions in the time-space matrix, all governed by the usual laws of physics. The second is a non-physical realm occurring in an ephemeral "space" generated by specific manipulations of data flows which precisely mimic the processes known as logical operations. It is governed by semantic laws and, because it isn't physical, is not subject to physical laws. This point is fundamental:

The semantic realm does not exist in the time-space-matter-energy universe of physics. It therefore has no mass or energy of its own, meaning the laws of mass-energy do not apply.

In the manipulation of data flows by suitably designed switches, there is no leakage of energy. This is the quintessential point, the *sine qua non* of this model. The data impulses and the switches manipulating them consume energy but the logical functions they are performing do not. There is a total disjunct between the two. A set of switches that was not designed to underwrite logical functions will consume energy without carrying any informational content. Rearranging the switches will allow them to mimic specific truth tables but *they will not*

DOI: 10.4324/9781003183792-3

require extra energy to do so. The law of conservation of mass-energy remains intact: logical processing is therefore a very successful free-rider on a material mechanism. Without this distinction, there could be no duality. In the specifications of an informational realm, this is Design Constraint No. 1.

Design Constraint No. 2: the switching achieves *something,* but the outcome is independent of the physical mechanism. At present, we have no formal way of characterising what it achieves except in terms of the output. A set of inert switches with no data flow does nothing; once data are channelled through them, something is achieved. The data are manipulated and, depending on the settings, a sonnet pops out, or perhaps the design for a new type of bullet. Critically, the informational content of the output does not affect the energy used by the switches in the process. The logic gates are themselves entirely neutral to the content of the information they are manipulating. There is *no relationship between the informational content and the physical state of the gates,* meaning information cannot be reduced to, identified or equated with, its material substrate.

For psychiatry, this means mind can never be reduced to or explained away as brain [1]. Brain is the *mechanism* of mind, but it is not the mind itself. A full knowledge of a physical brain can never explain the informational or mental content of that brain. Similarly, the physical state of every computer leaving a factory is known in enormous detail. It is not possible for a person who knows the detail, however minutely, to make any meaningful predictions about what content will be coded into that computer's memory even one hour after its new owners start to use it. The physical state does not determine the semantic state and, for any universal computing device, never can. *A fortiori*, this is true of the human brain and would remain true even if we knew its codes, which we don't, and possibly never will.

Design Constraint No. 3: What goes on between input and output is non-physical; it is nonetheless real. For want of a better term, we can call the *process* of data manipulation an informational space. Note how I have mixed the terms: there is, of course, no space involved, it is purely conceptual, an attempt to grasp an idea so slippery that many highly intelligent people have decided it is either impossible, self-contradictory - or self-deception. In Gilbert Ryle's terms, it is actually an "informational non-space" [2]. Nonetheless, this metaphorical space is a real thing. I can change it by installing new information to give a different outcome or I can change the switching process while leaving the outcome un-affected: $(A \rightarrow B)$ is logically equivalent to $\neg(A \wedge \neg B)$ and to $(\neg A \vee B)$. The rules governing the basic process of data manipulation are functionally equivalent to Boole's *Laws of Thought.*

An immaterial information space functions as a real entity by virtue of its ability to act upon the natural world, yet it does so without breaching the laws of thermodynamics. That is, it constitutes a novel form of "real," one that emerges from but is *not part of* (is ontologically distinct from) the physical realm. It is therefore legitimate to speak of the physical realm and of the informational realm because they are governed by entirely distinct sets of laws: for that reason alone, they are "two incommensurable orders of being." To complete the description, an informational space is most emphatically rule-governed. Therefore, there is no magic element involved, no miracles, it is not "...so mysterious that it keeps science at bay forever" (Dennett). It is a rational phenomenon that emerges just by the action of data switching by certain very tightly specified physical devices. If there is no switching, such as in trees and rocks, no informational space can be generated, so trees and rocks don't have/can't have mental properties. Thus, this model positively excludes the ancient idea that trees and other inanimate objects can have spirits or such like (for more on emergence, see Sect.5.2).

By the same argument, DNA does not itself *generate* an informational space. It is part of the mechanism that carries coded information which a suitably equipped reader (RNA) can use, but it has no switching capacity of its own. Thus, DNA is no more capable of generating an informational space than the pages of this book or the hieroglyphs carved into the walls of an ancient Egyptian funerary chamber. They *carry* codes but they are themselves completely in-sentient. They have no data flow and do not manipulate information in any way. In fact, the whole point of encoded information, especially DNA, is that it *doesn't* change. A text book whose pages changed overnight may have a place in a Harry Potter school but it wouldn't be much use elsewhere (except, perhaps, in eco-nomics). As part of this, there are elaborate intracellular mechanisms whose function is to prevent changes to the DNA code, to eliminate damage or var-iation. That is the very antithesis of the concept of switching which is based on the capacity of the device to change its settings, as it were.

Design Constraint No. 4: With certain caveats, it is not just any switching that can generate a suitable informational space, it has to be precisely coherent. It has to reproduce the specific pattern of input-output relationships of the known logical operators. Could there be other operators, say on a different planet, or maybe in creatures like the octopus? We can't answer that but we can certainly say that "mere switching" is not enough. Thus, despite the prodigious rate of switching that takes place in a working telephone exchange, its activity is in-coherent so the exchange will never have a mental life of its own. Switching is the essential operation and is independent of its medium; therefore, it is conceivable that machines could generate informational states which would be functionally indistinguishable from our own mental states. Just as Turing predicted [3].

A physical disturbance of the switching mechanism is likely to interfere with its performance, thereby degrading the informational space, but the output of an informational space depends on more than just the physical integrity of its logic gates. It also depends on the quality of the input data set and the validity of the algorithms by which the data are manipulated. That is, degraded performance of the informational space does not imply a physical cause. It is at just this point that the entire program of biological psychiatry runs into the sand.

In this model, it also follows that disembodied information is impossible, so ghosts and spirits, telepathy and prescience, auras, crystals and meridians of energy, etc. go back to the fairy stories where they belong. This has direct sig-nificance for psychiatry as it's not so long since people believed that mental disorder was caused by demonic possession (unfortunately, there are still some who do). Very often, this led to the most brutal and depraved mistreatment of the mentally-troubled. The biocognitive model positively excludes the belief system that spawned such crimes.

3.2 Mind as an informational space

Is the mind an informational space? Firstly, Table 3.1 compares the parameters of Descartes' thinking thing and the concept of an informational space, as derived above.

Given his "design specifications," Descartes couldn't prevent people saying that his *res cogitans* was just tricked up magic. On the other hand, the concept of an informational space is defined such that it positively excludes all supernatural connotations. It is dualist, because an informational space is not governed by the laws of the physical universe (and vice versa) but it is entirely a natural or non-magical dualism.

So is the mind an informational space? To answer this question, we have to specify precisely what we mean by mind. I will follow the model outlined by philosopher, David Chalmers (b. 1966), whose concept of a natural dualism has attracted a lot of attention since it was published nearly twenty-five years ago [4]. Chalmers writes: Consciousness exists as a real, non-physical thing which arises from the brain's activity by certain psychophysical laws, or laws of supervenience, which we can understand. Note that he said consciousness, not mind. Even though it's all the rage these days, the word consciousness is poorly-defined. Its appeal lies in sounding just that bit more scientific than "mind," although it doesn't convey anything more than the common word. However, it doesn't give any clues as to the various functions called "unconscious mental events," so I prefer to avoid it. Nonetheless, it leads to the soundbite so closely associated with Chalmers' name, the concept of "the hard problem of consciousness." This needs a bit of explanation.

Modern neurophysiology has revealed that many brain functions are entirely physiological in nature. Functions such as control of plasma osmolality, regulation of the pituitary hormones, central control of temperature and respiration, etc, are localised in the brain but still work in a person who is otherwise "brain

Table 3.1 Comparison of Descartes' *Res Cogitans* and Conceptual Informational Space

Criterion	Descartes	Informational Space
Utterly different from material matter	✓	✓
Exists independently of material matter	✓	X
Unextended, unlocalised	✓	✓
Invisible to all physical forces	✓	✓
Causally effective	✓	✓
Infinite output	✓	✓
Consistent with laws of thermodynamics	X	✓

dead." These are neurological functions which occur in the brain as a matter of anatomy, and don't form part of the mind as the term is normally used. As they don't represent any conceptual problems, we can leave them aside.

The class of "mental events" concerns all those functions that we normally call "mental," such as deciding, acting, perceiving, recalling, feeling, emotion etc. It is immediately clear that the set of all mental functions divides in two groups, those Chalmers called the psychological, meaning the informational and executive functions, and the experiential, meaning those related to ineffable experience. Without making any anatomical claims, his model of mind is functionally of two parts, or bicameral.

The first room in his two-room apartment holds all the knowing and decision-making processes that form the basis of our actions. These include what we know, such as our accumulated knowledge, our beliefs, plans, hopes, ambitions etc; what we decide from moment to moment; communication, including speech and knowledge gained from the senses; memory, and others. The second room is the very obvious "internal TV" of the classic senses (vision, cutaneous sensation, taste, etc), as well as emotions and a variety of other rather poorly understood but very important senses such as balance, spatial location etc. Unfortunately, when people talk of "consciousness," they may mean any one or all, of one or both parts of this very broad group of functions. To avoid any problems, I will use the word "mind" to mean all of the above, i.e. everything that would normally be considered mental in nature.

3.3 Informational functions of mind

The first group comprises the informational functions. These represent no conceptual difficulties for a materialist theory of mind. These days, machines routinely make decisions based on highly complex information, so our search for a non-magical, non-circular account of mind is off to a good start. In fact, so is a non-mentalist psychology because the essential point of all our informational processes is that they are out of sight of the eye of introspection. I don't know how I make decisions, I simply make them. Try this little experiment: Lift up your right arm. Did you catch yourself in the act of making that decision? Try it again, and again, but you will never be able to apprehend the instant at which you "choose" to do it. The act of deciding is forever silent, hidden from awareness but it is still real and it is entirely your decision. You can't plead 'not guilty' on the basis that you can't recall making the decision to act, because all those decisions are inaccessible, including the act of deciding to plead "not guilty."

Most of the decisions we make each day do not involve any conscious deliberation. The principal features of the executive or knowing part of mental life - Chalmers' psychological mind - are that it is very fast, it is silent and it is communicable. For example, I hear you speaking: without any sense of effort or delay, I understand exactly what you are saying. Similarly, while speaking, I do not know what will be the third next word that I will use but it will be contextually appropriate, it will be pronounced correctly and you will understand it instantly. I am not able to apprehend the processes by which these decisions are made, they are forever unknowable. This is part of what is meant by "unconscious decision-making."

These features apply without exception to all decisions we make. We don't know how we know this thing is an apple but the knowledge is there as soon as we see it. We don't know why we think something is funny, the decision is made for us and we are helpless to prevent it (as a medical student, I was incapable of not laughing at the professor's mistakes, which is never a good start to a medical career). I am scrambling down a rocky slope, jumping from rock to rock without any suggestion that I am "thinking about" what I am doing, my body makes that decision for me and I don't stumble. I am driving my wagon along a rocky, winding bush track, changing gears several times per minute, braking and accelerating as needed, all without any awareness of making the myriad decisions that keep the vehicle upright and moving. Something starts to fall and I reach out to stop it; there is no thought of "what I need to do," I just do it. A ball is thrown to me; I run then jump and catch it, without any consideration of the science of ballistics. But monkeys can do most of this, and dogs. As Descartes understood perfectly, there is nothing in principle that could be called "magic" about decisions. To account for the very great bulk of human behaviour, all we need is a powerful decision-making organ in the head, and the job is done. We can call this organ a "data-processor" or "calculator" or "computing device" without making any assumptions as to how it actually works.

All our knowledge of neurophysiology indicates that the brain functions as a high-speed, modular data processor, able to take a wide variety of informational inputs and formulate an outcome faster than we can apprehend - fast enough to save our lives. Conceptually, this is a pushover. Shannon's concept of switches as Boolean logic devices gives the basis for a materialist model of decision-making. In principle, the process is not complex. The eye perceives a sign, say a dot of green light on a black background. This triggers a volley of impulses in the optic nerve which travel back to the brain via a series of processing points or nuclei in the brain stem. The ensuing data flow is then sent to the visual cortex of the brain, located in the occipital region at the rear of the skull. After further processing and interaction with other inputs, a final signal is dispatched to activate, say, the right forefinger.

In this simple example, information flows from retina to brainstem to cortex, then down the spinal tract to the spinal motor neurons which act upon the motor endplate of the effector muscles. The data flow remains in exactly the same form throughout, as action potentials in neurons. It does not change at any point. The only change is when its significance changes. Some neurons act only as conduits for passing signals from one part of the body to another, the sort of thing that brought out the engineer in Shannon. However, in the brain itself, and not open to anything we could call 'conscious introspection,' the nerve impulses are processed according to the rules of a dual-valued calculus, Boole's Laws of Thought. *Their significance changes even though their physical nature is unchanged*. That point is crucial.

Consider the example above. The instructions given to the student participating in the study are:

> If the light is green and today's date is an even number, press button A.
> If the light is red and it is an odd-numbered day, press button B.
> In all other cases, do nothing.

The instructions are coded into the brain in such a form that activating them results in a volley of nerve impulses. These interact with the incoming impulses from the retina, via a system of functional logic gates built into the neurons themselves, to activate just one behavioral outcome out of the infinite repertoire of possible responses such as "Stand on your head in the corner."

It is exactly what Turing and all the early pioneers of the IT revolution had in mind when they said we would soon talk of computers as thinking and deciding. In Chalmers' expression, knowledge and executive decisions constitute the 'easy problem of consciousness.' However, we can expand the notion a little for the purposes of human behaviour.

3.4 Modularity

My use of the term "modular" in relation to the brain may cause some concern. It was introduced into cognitive sciences by the philosopher Jerry Fodor (1935–2017) in his 1983 book, *Modularity of Mind* [5]. Fodor was closely associated with the linguist Noam Chomsky (b. 1928), who, over many years, has developed and expanded the concept of an innate "language module." As much as we can admire Chomsky's social and political writings, it is often the case that his technical works lack the same elegance and precision [e.g. 6]. He appears to suggest that until about 60,000 years ago, *H. sapiens* had no capacity for language. Suddenly, as a result of some mutation, a "faculty of language" arose, presumably in one fortunate but fecund individual, and then spread to endow the rest of us. If that is what he is saying, it is impossible. Linguist Vyvyan Evans (b. 1968) has mounted a detailed case against the notion [7], strongly supported from a different approach by Daniel Everett (b. 1951) [8].

Fodor's use of the term "module" was originally applied to language, in the sense of a singular function, uniquely realised in a dedicated part of the brain, isolated from and unaffected by the workings of other modules. Both Everett and Evans have shown that language simply does not meet these criteria; indeed, nothing else does, either. In this sense, the idea is an artefact. When I use the term "modular," I mean that the brain can attend to a variety of different functions at the same time without them interfering with each other – well, within limits. Thus, I can talk to you while walking down a flight of stairs, at the same time as reaching into my pocket to find my keys and nodding a greeting to somebody who passes us on the stairs. Probably the expression "multi-channel processor" is more appropriate.

A simple example will show how the concept of genetically-determined, mental/cerebral modules is misdirected: swimming. It is the case that humans can swim. Not all learn, but most Australians can. That doesn't mean we have a genetically-based "swim module" hard-wired into our Antipodean heads which arose as a spontaneous mutation a few hundred years ago. What it means is that, because of the combination of a specific gravity below one (about 0.98), combined with mobile paddles on each corner of our bodies, *and* the ability to hold our breath at will, we can comfortably propel ourselves through water without immediately drowning (but so can rats, they are very good at swimming underwater). Each of those features is under entirely separate genetic control. It is the combination of these unrelated biological factors, similar to what Evans calls "an amalgam of various mental competences" [7, p. 240] that leads to the performance of swimming. In this sense, swimming is an emergent capacity (see Chap 5): nothing about our DNA says we have to swim but, if we choose, we can learn how to combine our mental competences.

Thus, we have abilities which are composed of a variety of different functions, arising from different brain regions, that give what appears to be a novel performance. That doesn't mean the performance is genetically-based as an entity, only that our brains are well-equipped with a broad range of subroutines that can be combined in near-infinite ways. Language combines passably good hearing with very fine tone discrimination; good short-term memory; conceptual memory and processing, and very fine control of breathing, larynx, lips and tongue (very few animals can move their whole tongue side to side, as distinct from licking around a corner, as cows do). It is absolutely impossible for all these functions to arise at once by a single or even hundreds of mutations. We do not have a language module, or language acquisition device, or faculty of language as such. Language developed slowly over perhaps 50,000 generations until it reached its modern level with early modern humans. Neanderthals could certainly speak.

3.5 Logic gates and neurons

Behaviour is rule-governed but the rules function behind the scenes, as it were. Indeed, we may not even be able to say what they are but they are real nonetheless. This is seen in language acquisition, when children learn to speak in grammatically correct languages without anybody telling them the rules, and even without their being able to verbalise any of the rules. Often, their errors are highly revealing, as every parent knows:

I seed the man.
I are wanting icecream.
You wetted me.

In adult behavior, rules may be explicit or implicit, and many significant beha-vioral rules may even have been acquired preverbally. Individuals may have lots of rules or hardly any; they may be internally consistent or inconsistent; they may mesh with the rules of the larger society, ignore them or contradict them. Any decision may involve just one or two rules, or many; decisions can be influenced moment to moment by changing circumstances with the result that people may appear rigid one moment, and vacillating the next. Where do these rules reside in the brain? I don't know but there is little doubt that certain parts of the brain are critical in integrating information and rules from a variety of sources.

As background, there are some 86 billion cortical neurons in the brain, of which 69 billion are in the cerebellum, dedicated to motor control. This means that the process of holding a human body upright as it reaches for its mobile phone while bounding down stairs is amazingly complex. No wonder it is taking engineers so long to make a general purpose robotic housemaid. Of the re-maining 17 billion cortical neurons, many more are dedicated to motor activity, which leaves only about 12 billion for making decisions and all other mental functions such as perception. Each cerebral neuron can have up to 10,000 connections, so the possibilities are fairly substantial. If each neuron functions as a microprocessor with, say, one logic gate per connection, then we have some-thing of the order of 120,000,000,000,000 (120trillion, or $1.2.10^{14}$) logic gates dedicated to higher cortical functions (executive and perceptual functions) in each human brain. This is a very large number.[1]

Currently, the international IT industry produces about 400trillion logic gates a month. That's for all the computers, phones, tablets, satellites, planes, ships, cars, TVs toys, fridges, factories, hospitals, universities, for all military forces, the stu-pefying capacity of the national security state, and so on, that we use in this age of information. That is, in one year, the entire worldwide IT industry can only pro-duce the computing power of 36 humans at the most. If, however, there are ten or even a hundred logic gates per neuronal connection, the final total could be something like 12 quadrillion (10^{15}) logic gates functioning as the processing mechanism for human mentation. This suggests that, if anything can, the human brain can generate an informational space to satisfy the conditions shown in Table 3.1. This gives us an entree to Chalmers' "hard problem of consciousness."

3.6 Hard problem of consciousness

Behaviorists, as you will recall, tried to write the mind out of their explanation of behaviour. British philosopher Sir Alfred Ayer reputedly said that to be a

---

1 Consider an even larger number. The surface area of 86billion neurons is about 22,000m². There are about 3,000 Na$^+$ channels per square micrometer, or 3.10^{15} psm. Thus, the total Na$^+$ channels per brain is of the order of 66.10^{18}, an impossibly high number. If each logic gate has even 100 channels, we are talking of a cosmic number of gates in the brain, and therefore almost incomprehensible feats of calculation. The mysterians may yet win.

behaviorist was to pretend to be anaesthetised from the neck up. What he meant was that there is something real that takes place in the head, even if we can't see it in the laboratory. I look at the sky and there is an experience we call blue. There is nothing blue inside my brain, of that I am sure, but the sensation of blueness cannot be gainsaid. For Chalmers, explaining the *experience* of blue, or of pain, or of fear, constitutes the difficult part of the problem of consciousness.

A lot of philosophers claim that it doesn't need to be explained. Daniel Dennett tries to brush off this kind of phenomenon, saying that pain, for example, is nothing to get excited about. If he steps on your foot, he says, you will feel only a fleeting pain which is so minor as not to warrant the label of "suffering." It would, he says, be a "risible" misuse of the term to apply it to an irritation that is no more than "...a brief, negatively-signed experience... of vanishing moral significance" [9, p220]. A brief experience is not the same as no experience; vanishing moral significance is not of no significance. A brief rape is not the same as no rape. Perhaps he also believes the pain of torture is "of vanishing moral significance" but it is unlikely he has ever tried it. Clearly, Dennett is not trying to explain conscious experience, he is trying to explain it away which is, at best, a profoundly dubious move.

The phenomena, the experiences, the qualia, etc, which are part of being an alert, aware, sentient being, are genuinely something, some *thing* we need to explain, not to explain away. Torture is no laughing matter. An orgasm is something that boredom is not. To claim otherwise, to try to airbrush them away, is to pretend to be anaesthetised from the neck up - and down.

The neurons of the brain's motor and physiological systems work in a computational mode, of that we can now be sure (I don't want to restrict the term yet, the computation may be analogue or digital, it doesn't matter; see Sect. 4.6). It is not feasible to suggest that the neural systems which serve as the mechanism of conscious experience, systems based in neurons which are physiologically exactly the same as the rest of the brain, do not also function in the computational mode. In the absence of any other remotely plausible explanation, we can accept *pro tem* the following assertion:

> *Conscious experience arises by virtue of the brain's capacity to operate as a high-speed data processor. The specific microarchitecture of the brain is necessary to generate conscious experience. Applied within that architecture, acquired rules are sufficient.*

These features have the potential to resolve the "hard problem of consciousness." Note that I didn't say "human brain." Apes have practically the same visual system as we do, and they respond to colour and movement exactly as we do; therefore, by Occam's razor, they see exactly as we do, or so close it doesn't matter. The same is true of many other animals: the notion that we humans alone have something unique called conscious experience is not worth pursuing. So, because there aren't as many spare neurons in an ape's brain compared with ours, whatever generates conscious experience doesn't require vast computing power *and* it has been around for a long time. Did dinosaurs see red? Birds can discern colours and sounds with great precision, so I'm sure dinosaurs could, or something similar.

To recapitulate, the biocognitive model says that, in addition to its executive functions, part of the brain's data-processing capacity generates another informational space of a unique kind. It is separate from but intimately related to the informational space called the knowledge realm. It doesn't require a lot of computing hardware (or wetware, in brain terms) so it must involve some very clever but subtle processing. Evidence for conscious experience is widespread in nature and is therefore old in evolutionary terms.

Somehow, the two parts of this informational space act upon each other to generate the illusion and the knowledge of something that doesn't exist in nature, such as blue. Nature doesn't have colour; by some subtle recursive activity, the visual system manufactures the sense we call colour but it is constrained within the individual brain's informational space, and is thus wholly private and ineffable. Why colour and not something else? Why do ears hear, tongues taste and fingers feel? The different sensory organs capitalise on the energy forms for which they are specialised. The visual system carries a vast amount of information per millisecond, about 2000 times as much as the aural system, and gives a very accurate impression of what is "out there." We use our eyes to find food, not our ears. Tickles are poorly localised, pain much more so. Each sensory system maximises the unique impact of its particular energy form to give us a highly detailed impression of the world we move in.

But why *colour*? Why *sound*? There are two responses here. First, I don't know, but I suspect the actual sensations as we experience them have a lot to do with memory. It may be that the path into memory is via these experiences, that memory can only accept certain sorts of information, but that's conjecture. Second, the senses have to be very different; if it were not colour, it would be something else but it would be very different from smells. How do sharks and other animals experience electroperception? We don't know, but it won't be anything like the aroma of dead meat. How do birds know they are following the correct migratory paths? In another universe, could we all be zombies, apparently alive and functioning but with no inner experience? The answer to that is a qualified yes, but it doesn't affect this model because we're not talking about other universes.

Emotions are somewhat different as they are generated internally and then experienced by the same sorts of processes as external perception, except the receptors are also internal. Let's say that the amygdala has an important role in anger. I see something happen in front of me. Immediately, based on my implicit knowledge (rules) of what is right and wrong, I compute that this event is bad and ought not to happen. Signals are sent from the executive areas of the brain to the amygdala, activating it. This activity is then fed, directly or indirectly, back to the higher centres whereby that input, and that input alone, is experienced as the emotion of anger. Without the amygdala, I can have an intellectual awareness that something is bad but it will be abstract, with no sensation of anger to reinforce the message [10]. In this model, the subcortical emotional centres are triggered by the higher executive centres. Their activity is fed back to the cerebral cortex by a mechanism similar to that by which external perception reaches the cortex. Therefore, if I don't like experiencing certain emotions, I either have to work out my private rules that generate them, and change the rules involved, or I can change my external reality (like get a less troublesome job).

Conscious experience is an ephemeral artefact that is "manufactured" by the brain or, in modern terms, generated in real time by the brain's data processing capacity. However, it is not *witnessed* by a small person inside the head. Rather, as a person, I am the unique totality of my current ephemeral experiences. I am an illusion, a mirage unto myself assembled from the outputs of a diverse range of functioning modules. My sense of there being something compellingly real and continuous about being me is fragile, utterly dependent on the continued well-being of my neurons.

You can't access my private reality, nor I yours; while you may be a zombie, I'm sure I'm not. All I have to do is see the wonder of a brilliant blue sky, or feel the salty spray from a storm-driven swell, to know there is some *thing* called *me* - which is what Descartes said nearly 400 years ago. I know I'm real because I can walk to the window and open it: I have causal power over my surroundings. I am not reducible to my neurons because my language and other symbolic functions are explicitly irreducible: that's what symbol *means*. The expression *x symbolises y* means that *x* stands for or represents *y* but is not and never can be *y* itself. I am real to myself but you will never find me inside my head because I'm not that sort of real: I can see a green hillside but you will not find anything green inside my head. You just have to take my word for it: I know green grass when I see it, even under an orange light.

Using this model, the claim that there is only one sort of reality, the physical, material, matter-energy-time-space sort of reality, is out of date. If you want to be dramatic, you could almost say ghosts are back in vogue. Actually, make that "ghosts," as they're rather humdrum "ghosts" with no supernatural properties whatsoever. Worse still, they exist only insofar as the brains that generate them continue to do their job. I may know green when I see it but it's an illusion. My private experience is insubstantial but not supernatural; and death is final.

3.7 Mental disorder

Modern psychiatry denies the possibility of the mentality of mental disorder. As the opening quotations in Chapter 1.1 showed, orthodox psychiatry is determined to hammer mental disorder into a tight biological box. If a few tender bits don't quite fit, don't worry, the sharp edges of the modern diagnostic system will amputate them. There is, however, an alternative view. In briefest terms, if the human mind is an emergent informational state, then primary errors can and will arise in that state, independently of the physical state of the switching device (brain) that generates the informational state. Primary errors can arise either because the input data set is faulty, or because the processing algorithms are faulty, or both. The mere fact that we are information processors (hardly in dispute these days) does not protect us against making mistakes; indeed, it opens entirely new vistas of error, as everybody who uses a computer knows too well. It is simply not the case that all errors in human mental life are biological errors.

Nobody knows how much money has been spent on biological research in psychiatry over the past sixty years but, in modern terms, it would be approaching $150billion. In all that time, and despite all the hype of the drug industry, nothing significant or consistent has been found concerning the nature of mental disorder. Not even a single mental disorder has ever been shown to have a basis in disordered brain physiology. Biological psychiatry scuttles along behind general medical research, picking up the latest high-tech tools as they are developed and finding a plethora of minuscule changes in the brain that are trumpeted as "a major breakthrough in the search for the cause of mental disorder." Not one of the so-called "discoveries" has ever amounted to anything. Not one of them has led to an improvement in the lot of the mentally disturbed. Today's hot findings don't become tomorrow's background knowledge, as happens in general medicine, they are simply forgotten, erased from the collective memory, as recalling them is too embarrassing. Who today remembers biogenic amines? Taraxein? Minimal brain damage? Don't worry, they were just dumb ideas floated by excitable academics, we've come so far since then.

If they had just stayed thought balloons, it wouldn't have mattered but they didn't. As soon as an idea gains currency, somebody rushes out to apply it to the mentally-troubled. Who could forget the lobotomy? Insulin coma therapy? Deep sleep therapy? Well, a lot of psychiatrists are doing their best to forget those things ever happened because now they've got the Chemical Imbalance of the Brain. The best part of the chemical imbalance trope is that it can never be proven wrong. If your research program doesn't find it, well that just goes to show it's a very subtle chemical imbalance which needs lots more expensive research. Reminding biological psychiatrists of all their previous disasters is seen as tasteless, a good way of ending a pleasant conversation.[2]

Bizarrely, the answer to the question of the nature of mental disorder has been sitting under our noses all along. Because psychiatry has been so determined to sterilise itself of any taint of "magical thinking," it has discarded the mind as a basis for a science. And in so doing, it threw out the possibility of establishing a new kind of science, one more in keeping with modern concepts of informational science as opposed to test tubes and bunsen burners, but a science nonetheless. Chemical imbalances are just so twentieth century.

The renowned science fiction writer, Arthur C Clarke, said: "Any sufficiently advanced technology is indistinguishable from magic." To a committed reductionist, a natural dualist theory of mind is "indistinguishable from magic," but that is an ideological stance, not scientific [11]. Going back to Newton's magical force field of gravity, my case is that the *mentality* of mental disorder is *not* "...so

---

2 For a very scary night, watch *The Lobotomist* on PBS Frontline.

great an Absurdity that… no Man who has in philosophical Matters a competent Faculty of thinking can ever fall into it." Instead, it is the future of psychiatry.

References

[1] McLaren N (2007). Brain disease, mental disease, and the limits to biological psychiatry. Chapter 2 in *Humanizing Madness: Psychiatry and the Cognitive Neurosciences*. Ann Arbor, Mi.: Future Psychiatry Press.

[2] Ryle G (1949). *The Concept of Mind*. London: Hutchinson. Reprinted Penguin University Books, 1973.

[3] Turing AM (1950). Computing machinery and intelligence. *Mind*. 59: 433–460.

[4] Chalmers DJ (1996). *The Conscious Mind: in search of a fundamental theory*. Oxford: University Press.

[5] Fodor J (1983) *Modularity of Mind*. Cambridge, MA: MIT Press.

[6] Chomsky (2002) *New Horizons in the Study of Language and Mind*. Cambridge: University Press.

[7] Evans V (2014). *The Language Myth: why language is not an instinct*. Cambridge: University Press.

[8] Everett DL (2017) *How Language Began: the story of humanity's greatest invention*. New York: Norton/Liveright Publishing.

[9] Dennett DC (1991). *Consciousness Explained*. London: Penguin Books (1993).

[10] Sapolski RM (2017). *Behave: The Biology of Humans at Our Best and Worst*. London: Bodley Head.

[11] McLaren N (2013). Psychiatry as Ideology. *Ethical Human Psychology and Psychiatry* 15: 7–18.

4 Toward a formal basis for a theory of mind

The positivists have a simple solution: the world must be divided into that which we can say clearly and the rest, which we had better pass over in silence. But can anyone conceive of a more pointless philosophy, seeing that what we can say clearly amounts to next to nothing?

If we omitted all that is unclear we would probably be left with completely uninteresting and trivial tautologies.

Werner Heisenberg (1901–1976)

Every great and deep difficulty bears in itself its own solution. It forces us to change our thinking in order to find it.

Niels Bohr (1885–1962)

Behind it all is surely an idea so simple, so beautiful, that when we grasp it – in a decade, a century, or a millennium—we will all say to each other, how could it have been otherwise? How could we have been so stupid?

John Archibald Wheeler (1911–2008)

4.1 Defining information: preliminaries

Given that the concept of information is of crucial importance to the model – we could almost say its justification – what can be said about information itself? What *is* this thing called information? The first point to note is that for a bio-logical reductionist, the notion of information is a pushover. In the final analysis, they say, everything is just molecules and chemicals sloshing around in the dark: If you want to know the nature of information, just look at the nature of matter and energy: there's the answer, so where's your problem?

If, however, we claim that the dualist nature of the universe rests on the idea of information *not* being reducible to physical matter, then we need to do better than that. Trouble is, however we approach the question, we seem to run into in-tractable problems, as philosopher Luciano Floridi (b. 1964) glumly concluded:

The concept of information has become central in most contemporary philosophy. However, recent surveys have shown no consensus on a single,

DOI: 10.4324/9781003183792-4

unified definition of semantic information. This is hardly surprising. Information is such a powerful and elusive concept... [1]

His more recent primer on information [2] offers descriptions of information at work but does not define it. Even his major work, entitled *The Philosophy of Information*, says only: "Information is still an elusive concept" [3, p30].

Robert Losee (b. 1952) emphasised how different people want different things from a definition of information:

> Electrical engineers wish to study the capacity of pieces of hardware and the physical connections between them. Linguists wish to understand how information is transmitted by languages and the nature of what lies at the core of communication. Mathematicians and computer scientists wish to study the processes by which software transforms input into output and the fundamental characteristics of transforming processes [4].

Losee, who is a professor of information (an informationist?), quoted other authors to illustrate some of the problems involved in this most abstract of notions:

> As Stonier reminds us, 'we must not confuse the detection and/or interpretation of information with information itself'... In an approach similar to defining information as meaning, information is often understood in terms of knowledge that is transmitted to a sentient being...

> Eventually, he arrived at what could be called the minimalist position but it lurches perilously close to the boundaries of science - or even straight across them:...'information is what remains after one abstracts from the material aspects of physical reality' (Resnikoff, 1989). The information in a structure is an immaterial ghost that co-exists with the physical object about which it informs.

> Normally, science prefers not to treat with immaterial ghosts, let alone assign them the crucial role in human affairs that information has held since the IT revolution. Fred Dretske (1932–2013) was similarly inclined:...it is common among cognitive scientists to regard information as a creation of the mind, as something we conscious agents assign to, or impose on, otherwise meaningless events. Information, like beauty, is in the mind of the beholder [5].

But can science deal with such subjective phenomena? Well, engineers can. As noted in Chapter 1, Claude Shannon was very careful to say what can be *done* with information but not what it *is*:

> The fundamental problem of communication is that of reproducing at one point either exactly or approximately a message selected at another point. Frequently the messages have meaning; that is, they refer to or are correlated

according to some system with certain physical or conceptual entities. These semantic aspects of communication are *irrelevant* to the engineering problem [6, emphasis added].

Essentially, Shannon was concerned with how to shove data into a tube while ensuring that what emerged at the other end accurately recreated what had gone in. As an engineer, he was not concerned with the content that went into the tube, be it philosophy or pornography; for engineers, nothing has really changed since 1948. The entire IT revolution has been based on the notion of what you can do with information (and how much money you can make from it), not on the idea of what information actually *is*. Wolfgang Lenski [7] was perfectly clear on this point:

> Shannon's theory defines a way to measure information, it does not explain what it is.

It must not be forgotten that Shannon's seminal paper was entitled *A Mathematical Theory of Communication*, not of information. This raises an important question: If, as a pioneer of the information revolution, Shannon didn't/ couldn't define information, how did he know that what he was measuring was indeed information? The answer is that he didn't know and was hardly concerned. Although he knew the electrical impulses coursing through his circuits could potentially be used to convey meaning, or information, he was measuring impulses only: *there are impulses without meaning, but there is no meaning without impulses*. All too often, the revolutionary point of Shannon's work is not appreciated: by recognising that the vehicle is *not* the content, by splitting the physical from the non-physical, he commoditised information as just a matter of blips coursing through a channel, thereby helping unleash the IT revolution.[1]

> But there is indeed more to information than blips and, on this point, Losee offered......a general definition of information: Information is produced by all processes and it is the values of characteristics in the processes' output that are information.

Later in the paper, he rephrased this to read:

> Information may be understood as the value attached or instantiated to a characteristic or variable returned by a function or produced by a process [4].

As a definition, this must fail, as it begs the question (i.e. it assumes the truth of that which needs to be proven or explained). Value is itself an informational

---

1 For a brief historical review, see Seising [8]; he gives due credit to the Soviet mathematician, Andrei Kolmogorov. Erico Guizzo gives a readable background on these aspects of Shannon's ideas [9].

term: in order to explain "value," you assume or rely on a prior explanation of information. Thus, we can't use the idea of value to explain information.

4.2 Defining information

Losee's review shifts the emphasis away from physical engineering toward immaterial meaning, although I don't think his definition helps us much. But don't underestimate the influence of physicalists. Emboldened by their success, and drawing support from a small bunch of strident philosophers, they are trying to convince everybody that there is nothing mysterious hidden in the blips, that the engineering says it all. Their reason is the general trend over the past century to avoid anything that appears mentalist, on the erroneous basis that it necessarily is, or is tainted by, magical thinking (eg. [10]). That is, by ignoring the problem of the knowledge embedded in their flows of information, they are hoping it will go away. It won't. Like pressing on a water bed to get rid of a bump, it just pops up elsewhere, as in: "What is the nature of the physical brain that it can apprehend purely conceptual terms such as value?"

Consider my little Kindle ebook reader, which now holds a hundred and fifty books but weighs no more than the day I bought it. Yes, it is indeed physically different from the reader that arrived in the box as its memory has been re-organised according to instructions beamed from the far side of the planet. Every time I download a new book, the memory is adjusted to create a facsimile of the book. Just so, the reductionists chortle: surely that proves that at base, information is no more than tiny physical changes. But not so fast: these physical changes are the *mechanism* used to convey and store the information, but they are not the information itself. We could have the same book coded in a different form in another manufacturer's e-reader or, quaintly, on paper.

The changes in each memory cell are not random, they are highly specific. They are organised by a very specific and highly organised process called "language," which is designed to convey a predetermined code representing symbols that can only be accessed by people who know the code (in the case of this book, English speakers). It is not just a case of physical changes (in the e-reader) induced by other physical changes (in somebody's brain) because that initiates an infinite regress. Infinite regresses are never explanatory, they simply delay the day of reckoning. Physicalist explanations of information therefore fail. However, physicalists will gleefully point out that any attempt at a non-physical definition of information will inevitably beg the question, i.e. it will assume the truth of information in order to define itself.

As a first step, this isn't always bad: starting with Edward Jenner, physicians assumed the truth of the immune system long before they had the faintest clue how it worked. But is it possible to be rid of the circularity? Let's start with this working definition:

Definition 4.1. Information is an *assessment* of some *discernible* aspect of the universe by an entity with the *capacity* to *represent* states of affairs in a *symbolic calculus*.

Each of the words in italics presupposes some sort of mentalist ability, meaning it can only be explained in mentalist terms (the remaining nouns - universe, entity, affairs – are givens of the material universe and don't require explanation). An *assessment* is not a physical property. It is an action performed when one entity records certain points about another in a *symbolic* form. Yes, the features are recorded as tokens inscribed on a physical medium but the information the tokens represent (their signal value) is not the same as the token itself, and is independent of the medium. The tokens in the symbol 'beer' are not wet and foaming. The information contained in that particular symbol is *abstracted* from the refreshing drink but only a being with informational-processing capacities can *know* that. The tokens are physical but *abstraction* is another circular term as it implies some quality of the subject has been isolated so that it represents or denotes the original entity, yet the symbol is not and never will be identical with that entity: that just is the definition of symbol. This action can only be performed by an entity with the *capacity* to *represent* states of affairs in a *symbolic calculus,* which means we're back where we started, needing information to explain information. The same will happen with each of the italicised words: information cannot be explained by reduction but nor, at this stage, can we arrive at an entirely non-physical, non-circular definition.

Things are not looking good. Physicalist accounts of information founder on the disjunct between an entity and the symbol used to denote it, while non-physicalist accounts seem to be dogged by circularity. But is this so bad? I don't think so. My case is that we live in a dualist universe, each of which has to be defined in its own terms. Every attempt to define matter, energy, space and time wholly in their own terms must bog down in circularity. Similarly, because it is ontologically different from matter-energy, information cannot be defined in terms of the physical realm, it can only be defined in terms of itself. This should not be surprising. As early as 1948, the eccentric mathematician, Norbert Wiener (1894–1964), stated flatly:

> The mechanical brain does not secrete thought 'as the liver does bile,' as the earlier materialists claimed, nor does it put it out in the form of energy, as the muscle puts out its activity. Information is information, not matter or energy. No materialism which does not admit this can survive at the present day [11].

This is a clear assertion that narrowly-defined materialism (aka physicalism) cannot give a full account of the universe as we now know it, although there was no firm proof in Wiener's little book. Also in 1948, Shannon understood that any attempt to account for the semantic content of information in terms of the matter-energy functions of its tokens is doomed on the basis that they are not related. That's what the dual in dualism *means* (that damned word again). Wiener didn't live to see his view gain wider acceptance; even when he died, most people still didn't understand what he had said. They could think only in terms of *either* "scientific matter and energy" *or* "all that magical nonsense." Their beliefs shaped their perceptions. Shannon's new view has had to fight prejudice, not facts, but is now slowly taking over just because it works and the other view doesn't. Thus, we can tentatively accept this frankly dualist definition to see how it stands in its context and how it is used in the real world.

4.3 Consequences of Definition 4.1

The *first* thing to note about Definition 4.1 is that, axiomatically, there is no disembodied information, no such thing as information which is not coded in a suitable physical medium. Because information is captured, processed, stored or transmitted only by a dedicated physical mechanism, this is a necessary truth, not contingent. There may be novel forms of information encoded in media we cannot yet conceive but, if the medium is physical, its contained information isn't magic.

The *second* point is that there is no medium of information *per se*. The actual tokens that denote the information are inscribed in some medium but the status of the semantic content of the tokens is paradoxical. On the one hand, it exists only insofar as the tokens exist, so we say the tokens are necessary for the informational content. However, the tokens themselves do not determine the information. An informational content is independent of its physical implementation, so the tokens are necessary but not sufficient for information to exist. Information itself, however, has no medium: as an informational state, it doesn't exist any*where*. It comes into being *as content alone*. There is no such thing as "information without content" or "pure information."

In human terms, this means the notion of "consciousness without content" or "pure consciousness" is meaningless. Information just is the medium, it represents itself so there is no consciousness without content. How can this be? My response is: that's what dualism means. If you can only conceive of information in terms of its being reducible to a physical medium, you have missed the point of the notion of dual realms of physical reality and non-physical reality. Most emphatically, information is not governed by the laws of the physical realm. However, and perhaps confusingly, *there is no information if there is not a reader to read it*. The meaning of a symbol doesn't reside in the tokens, it resides in effecting changes in another informational state. A sign on a path with no pedestrians induces no change, and its informational content is therefore zero. Until it is read, a sign is just a pretty pattern.

Third, as an *abstraction* or *representation* of physical reality, any and all interesting information about the physical realm can be wrong. The only information that can't be wrong is truism, which is not interesting as it adds nothing to our understanding of the universe. Granted, parts of the disciplines of mathematics and logic are truism, but that has a different goal.

Fourth, information from a variety of different media can be rendered in a standard code and can therefore be combined and manipulated by defined operations in a suitable processor, even though the media themselves are incompatible (such as sound and light). This is the foundation of intelligent or directed behaviour as we normally understand it.

Finally, as an abstracted quality and with a suitable medium, information can be collected, stored, processed and transmitted independently of its author and its referent, which is the basis of communication. This allows us to extend the investigation.

4.4 Formalising computation as the basis of mind

All too often within the framework of materialist science, "immaterial" is mistakenly equated with "supernatural" so, inevitably, the very concept of a non-material mind is reflexively rejected as primitive or mystical thinking. Over the past century, people have struggled to explain how the mind may, in fact, be seen as physical but, despite the loud claims of physicalists (eg [10]), the field remains wide open. Because of the failure of "materialist theories of mind" to progress, we need to develop a conceptual basis for a non-material theory of mind but this is not easy. The risk is that any such theory will breach the principle of conservation of mass-energy, specifically at the point of interaction between the physical brain and the non-physical mind.

If the laws of the material time-space-matter-energy universe are unable to provide a clue as to the nature of mind, then we need to look further. And in fact, that definition of materialism is inadequate. The physical universe consists of the elements of time, space, matter and energy *as well as* the informational states that may control them. This expands the definition of "material" in a material universe and gives the clue. If mind is an informational state, then we have a conceptual opening to solving the problem of an insubstantial mind in a material universe. To retain credibility, we should not range beyond the current technology but I believe it already allows us to model a workable solution to the nature of mind and its relation to the brain.

For philosopher David Chalmers, the mind is a natural phenomenon, not miraculous. By means of (as yet undefined) psychophysical laws, and as a natural consequence of its functional architecture, the causally efficacious mind arises from or supervenes upon the healthy, intact brain's data processing capacity. The essential notion is that, given any suitable computational capacity, informational functions will emerge, regardless of the particular physical structure of the system. In the case of the brain, those just are cognitive functions. This defines a dualist world but it is a *natural* dualism. Chalmers further divides the human mind in two distinct realms, the knowing or executive, and the experiential. As he points out, the idea of mechanical (natural, non-miraculous) decision-making is now woven into the fabric of our society: explaining decision-making is thus seen as the "easy problem of consciousness."

Even for this part, he argued, the concept of computation is critical:

> Perhaps no concept is more central to the foundations of modern cognitive science than that of computation. The ambitions of artificial intelligence rest on a computational framework, and in other areas of cognitive science, models of cognitive processes are most frequently cast in computational terms [12].

In explaining the existence and function of the mind, he proposes that two conditions must be met: *computational sufficiency*, i.e. that a specific computational structure will suffice for mental properties, and *computational explanation*, meaning that computation can account for cognition. Two questions, he says, are immediately apparent:

> What are the conditions under which a physical system implements a given computation?... What is the relationship between computation and cognition?

The first question, Chalmers suggested, is satisfied as follows:

> A physical system implements a given computation when the causal structure of the physical system mirrors the formal structure of the computation.

This is conceptually very close to Shannon's analogue of logic and circuits. In more detail, the input, internal and output states of the physical system are precisely related or mapped to the equivalent input, internal and output states of the computational operation. In simple systems, this amounts to an isomorphic relationship between the system and its associated higher-order process. In more complex systems, the requirement that the internal states are also isomorphic becomes otiose as there are too many ways a particular output can be achieved. Clearly, computational machines can be built of a wide range of materials with an unlimited range of mechanisms, so a specific output state can be realised in many different ways, or what is now termed "multiply realisable" (that's the adverb multip-ly, not the verb multi-ply). What counts is the precise relationship between the input and output states of the physical system and of the computation.
  Chalmers concluded:

> ...the essential idea is very simple: the relation between an implemented computation and an implementing system is one of isomorphism between the formal structure of the former and the causal (i.e. physical) structure of the latter. (Regarding) implementation..., a computation is simply an abstract specification of causal organization.

That is, as long as a physical machine performs certain operations which precisely parallel the elements of token manipulation in one or other computational operation, machines can perform complex computations. Without this performance, there could be no cognitive mechanisms, meaning the concept of a natural dualist theory of mind would be still-born. As would we.
  Chalmers does not, however, say anything about the *mechanism* by which the computation takes place. My proposal is that *the brain generates a computational capacity by virtue of its function as a high-speed switching device* (of course, it could also be a low-speed switching device but then it would take you a week to read this sentence). With several qualifications, this capacity constitutes the mechanism underlying cognitive activity, from which the human mind emerges.

It is not the case that just any switching device will do, it must be a very specific type. A computational capacity does not arise just because there is a great deal of switching going on somewhere; rather, the process of switching must meet a lengthy series of exacting criteria. The *sine qua non* is that the physical switches act upon a data flow in such a manner that their input-output relationships are isomorphic with the input-output relations of the truth tables of the known logical operators. This satisfies Chalmers' implementation criterion, as above:

> A physical system implements a given computation when the causal structure of the physical system mirrors the formal structure of the computation.

4.5 Defining a computational model of mind

Such a system constitutes the general computational basis of a model of mind. In the next two sections, the essential features of a natural dualist model of mind will be developed. Each step in the process has to be specified in detail so that there are no loose ends, no points at which a "miracle" is necessary to complete the causal chain. This is rather like specifying each and every enzymic step in a metabolic process, or the ineffably complex elements of the immune system.[2]

4.5.1 A *symbol* is a sustained physical mark or object which, by convention, denotes or represents within an *abstract realm* any entity, event or process, physical or abstract (i.e. a state of affairs), but which is not itself the physical mark or object: an object cannot symbolise itself (this is clearly circular because we can't define symbols without invoking conventions, which only occur in abstract realms, while the definition of abstract realms is not yet independent of the concept of symbols). A representation of a particular state of affairs is a *construct*.

4.5.2 A *proposition* is a declarative statement formed by strings of symbols which express the relationship between two constructs. A proposition can itself be represented by a further symbol.

This formalises the basis of communication, the transfer of information between entities. As Shannon argued, this is the end of the road for engineers. But, in psychiatry, we're interested in more than the mechanics, we want to come to grips with the concept of meaning.

4.5.3 Propositions can be divided into *meaningful* and *meaningless*. A *meaningful proposition* recreates in a separate abstract realm (in human terms, in the audience's mind) a more or less accurate *representation* (facsimile) of

---

2 I feel I need to apologise for what follows but the definitions are essential for the rest of this work, and I can't find a less burdensome way of presenting them. Each definition builds on what has gone before.

all or part of the abstract realm which constitutes the speaker's *mental state*. *Meaningless propositions* fail to convey a facsimile of the speaker's mental state as they don't follow the agreed rules (as in "What on earth is he saying?" "I've no idea, it doesn't make sense," or "We'd better find somebody who speaks his language").

4.5.4 A mental state can be communicated only by following precise rules accepted by speaker and audience (transmitter and receiver), or *language*, regarding the transmission of the propositions needed to reproduce the mental state. A language is a code accepted by transmitter (speaker) and receiver (audience) which can be transmitted (communicated) through a physical medium (such as air, light, cables etc) by means of agreed symbols.

This shifts the concept of meaning, away from the "mere mechanics" of communication, such as physical impulses in a cable or pressure changes in air, to some event in the audience's mental state which is triggered by those physical impulses. Meaning inheres in the audience's head, not in the physical medium between speaker and audience, or in the code they are using. However, before we can talk of mental states, we need to expand the notion beyond an instantaneous event such as a word or sign, to something longer-lasting, because that's basic to a sense of self. But the essence of a mental life is understanding how different states of affairs relate to each other, which requires a more powerful mechanism than mere communication.

4.5.5 A cluster of related meaningful propositions constitutes an *abstract structure*. An abstract or immaterial structure exists only in an abstract realm (again, the word *structure* is a metaphor; we really mean a non-structure).

4.5.6 An *operation* is the process of manipulating the *relation* between two propositions in an abstract structure using an agreed sequence of transformations. To avoid confusion, we will use the word "signs" to denote operations, and "symbols" to denote the objects or processes upon which the signs operate For example, in (1+1=2), the digits 1 and 2 are symbols, while the remaining four elements (known as *right* and *left brackets, plus* and *equals*) are signs. Signs tell the operator, such as you, what to do with the symbols, but only if you already know which particular operation the signs denote.

Note we are talking in general terms not specific. Baboons don't seem to have much interest in quadratic equations but they certainly understand the relationship between danger (say a prowling leopard) and the safety of a tree. But we're humans, and we communicate by language, so we'll continue with the goal of providing a formal basis for communication:

4.5.7 In *formal systems*, essentially mathematics and logic, the number of operations is restricted. The system of rules (operations) and symbols is known as a *formal language*. *Natural languages* are less formal, with a strong descriptive basis but, for any language…

a. *syntactics* is the relation between symbols in a formal structure (roughly, grammar);
b. *semantics* is the relation of symbols and their denotata (roughly, meaning); and
c. *pragmatics* is the relation between symbols and symbol-using agents.

Together, these three fields constitute *semiotics*, the theory of signs, symbols and meaning.

4.5.8 A *calculus* is any coherent and consistent set of rules governing operations on and between symbols in an abstract structure, either as single entities or as propositions.

4.5.9 A *logical operator* defines certain very specific relationships between propositions in an abstract structure, namely, those associated with the processes of valid inference.

4.5.10 A *logical calculus* is a *dual-valued (Boolean) calculus* using the accepted logical operators (as distinct from, say, arithmetic operators or common language operators) as the only possible operations. In Boolean logic, there are sixteen operators, most of which are rarely if ever used. Ordinary propositional logic normally uses six operators (*not*, *and*, *or*, *identity*, *material implication* and *biconditional*) which can duplicate the remaining operations.

4.5.11 *Computation* is therefore the manipulation of symbols in accordance with a predetermined calculus. Both the symbols *and* the calculus exist only as elements in *abstract structures*.

This gives us the basis for a dualist universe. It takes us beyond the "mere mechanism" of a physical structure, to the point where states of affairs can be represented and manipulated in a non-physical realm.

4.6 Computation in action: birds

Let's have a break from definitions to consider our path. Our goal is to define the essential elements in satisfying Chalmer's implementation criterion ("A physical system implements a given computation when the causal structure of the physical system mirrors the formal structure of the computation"). We need this in order to provide a basis for the idea that mentality supervenes upon the physical structure of the brain. That is, we need to specify in detail the abstract requirements that must be satisfied before *any* physical system can implement a computational process, and apply this to the brain. This is the *sine qua non* of a dualist account of mind. If we can't specify computation, and show how the brain could conceivably implement it, we haven't left the starting blocks.

There are, it is true, people who object to the idea that something called computation could carry the immense burden of explaining why a pain hurts, or a sense of nervous anticipation. We will look at some objections in Sect. 4.8 below, as well as one of the major opponents in Sect. 8.4, but, meantime, it is important to have an idea of the scope of the idea of computation.

Our home in the rural outskirts of Brisbane looks across paddocks and a creek to an extensive state forest and national park, so we have a lot of wildlife on our property. Two prominent members of our little community are pied butcher-birds (*Cracticus nigrogularis*) and magpies (*Gymnorhina tibicen*), both of which are renowned as glorious singers (they are actually choristers). They are carni-vores, with grasshoppers forming a large part of their diet, although they hunt differently. Mapgies stalk imperiously across the grass, flushing grasshoppers and other insects, whereas butcherbirds tend to wait in trees and catch their food on the wing, or swoop down silently. Before the rains arrive, the grass is parched and dry and grasshoppers are scarce, so the birds have trained us to feed them if they come to the verandah just after dawn.

Magpies are courteous creatures who stand in a line on the backs of the chairs, waiting for the food to be thrown to them. However, it can be a bit of a battle as the butcherbirds are fast and agile, and will grab the morsels of food thrown to the bigger birds. Watching them is quite remarkable. In less than a second, butcherbirds launch themselves like little feathered missiles, zooming up to two metres to intercept the food just before it reaches the magpies. Often, I will send a scrap in one direction to lure the butcherbirds away, then flick a piece to the magpies but that doesn't always work. The butcherbirds will catch theirs, then turn back and snatch the magpies' breakfast. Occasionally, they miss a piece. In a flash, they turn and chase it as it falls, catching it in time to pull out of a death dive a hand's breadth above the floor, and coast back to their perches to eat it. For that spectacular maneuvre, they fly about seven metres in perhaps two sec-onds (12.5 km/hr), including executing two high-speed $110°$ turns.

Consider the mathematics involved. Crouching intently, they watch my hand but they don't move until I let the food go. They do not *follow* the target, but fly at speed in a straight line to intercept their target on its curving course. Bearing in mind that a human brain weighs about 1400 gm, while the birds' brains weigh about six grams, no human could move as fast or as accurately as these cheerful little brigands. So what is the process that takes place in their small heads that tells their wings to beat at just this speed and in this particular direction so they can arrive at a particular point in space at the same instant as the food? Whatever it is, it will involve some process by which symbols representing the four dimensional space they have to navigate are manipulated in accordance with a pre-existing calculus. Because both the symbols and the calculus exist only as elements in an abstract structure, and without restricting ourselves, we can call it a computational process.

I don't believe the birds have much understanding of differential calculus, sufficient to allow them to work out exactly where their beaks should be to snatch the food. However, nor am I relying on it when I throw the food in a curved trajectory so it arrives at a particular point near the magpies' heads for them to catch it without falling over. I accept that the birds can see me just as I can see them; that they have "worked out" I am not a danger to them; and that they need only act in a particular way toward me to be fed, i.e. that they have conditioned me. In the very broadest sense of the word, all of this is computation in action, and it is restricted to the animal world. There is no sense of the word that would allow us to say that trees or rocks compute.

When a plant turns toward the sun (phototropism), when rain falls, when ice cracks a rock or an egg hatches, there is no computation involved at all. Those processes are purely physical, occupying a separate realm of discourse from that shown by the birds at my home. In all animals studied, including birds, the cerebellum is of a form that we recognise as suitable for high speed computations involving movement in four dimensions. It seems vanishingly unlikely that in implementing its two different mental functions, executive processes and experience, the brain relies on totally different neuronal processes, one of which we know in great detail, and the other we haven't even begun to suspect. Until somebody has a better suggestion, I will accept that *all cerebral neurons rely on the same cellular processes to implement the computations subserving the separate knowledge and experience functions,* according to the definition at pt **4.5.11,** above. The only difference lies in the algorithms by which the computations are implemented.

To end the story, every year, as soon as the rains arrive and the grasshoppers start to breed, the birds stop coming. Another point is that each season, the parent birds teach their young their tricks.

4.7 Computation and the hard problem of consciousness

Now we can start to look at how the process of computation can be implemented in a brain to satisfy the hard problem of consciousness. In humans, mental activity is generated by neuronal processes which define the dualist nature of mind: At base, what *is* the mind? This question is prior to and distinct from the questions: What is the structure of mind? What are the mental contents? How does it work to produce behaviour and experience?

4.7.1 Unlike all other cells in the body, neuronal activity consumes energy but produces nothing. The goal of the activity of a nerve cell is to return itself to *status quo ante.* An impulse travelling along a nerve fiber must leave no trace of its passage. This forms the basis of its ability to conduct data and then to process it. Since clusters of neurons are neutral to the content of their activity, they can act as switches.

4.7.2 Because of its neuronal architecture (specifically, the precise molecular and sub-cellular function of neurons and their structural relationships), the brain has a capacity as a *high-speed, multi-modal data switcher and processor.* By this specific function, it generates a *conceptual informational space.* This is the basis of mind.

4.7.3 Certain forms of switching mimic the input-output relations of logical operators, thereby constituting *Boolean switches.* As such, they generate the capacity for the manipulation of data, i.e. *neuronal data-switching constitutes the physical mechanism required to implement a computational model of mind.*

Now we have a formal mechanism that provides the "extra level" in a dualist universe. We build on this as follows:

4.7.4 The lowest level of data switching, before Boolean switches appear, is incapable of generating an effective output. Its output is noise, but there is nothing to hear as it is abstract "noise" in an insubstantial medium. It is only when the switching becomes coherent that it can generate symbols (sustained representations of entities or events), so that the abstract realm becomes an informational space which can be communicated.

4.7.5 The first symbols are necessarily elementary but, as they increase in number, their permutations increase exponentially, up to formal abstractions. Given the disjunct between physical neuronal functions (the *mechanism* of mind) and the information the neurons carry, there is thus a clear explanatory line from the physiology of basic neuronal function to the highest levels of human analytic and executive functions. This eliminates the circular element in Definition 4.1.

4.7.6 Empirically, there are two components to mind, the *experiential realm*, of conscious experience, and the *executive realm*, in which are made the decisions that produce coherent behaviour. Both realms are generated by computational processes implemented in the brain's neuroarchitecture, using identical physical mechanisms (neuronal spike discharges) but manipulated by different sets of rules.

4.7.8 The executive realm is not accessible to introspection; it operates silently and rapidly to make decisions to activate the body's effector organs, meaning behaviour. The products of decision-making are public in that they can be conveyed to others. Very often, we have no recollection of making a decision but it is real and personal nonetheless. The experiential realm (realm of conscious awareness etc) is manifest, private, causally ineffective and ineffable. Emotions are part of this realm.

By these steps, we arrive at a dualist model of mind which satisfies Chalmers' criteria, of consciousness supervening upon the physical structure of the brain by a law-like process. Note that this model positively excludes a physicalist or reductionist explanation of mind.

4.8 Computational model of mind

Computational models of mind attract a range of criticism. Michael Rescorla (b. 1975) summarised the various themes as follows:

A key task facing computationalists is to explain what one means when one says that the mind "computes". A second task is to argue that the mind "computes" in the relevant sense. A third task is to elucidate how computational description relates to other common types of description, especially neurophysiological description (which cites neurophysiological properties of the organism's brain or body) and intensional description (which cites representational properties of mental states) [13].

We can look at each of these tasks in turn. The first is easy: the mind does not compute. As an informational space, the mind is the *product* of a computational process which, in turn, it can influence by means of its own semantic content. Essentially, the mental contents tell the brain what to compute: the bird sees the food moving and instructs its cerebellum which path to compute. The computational process occurs at the neuronal level, not at the level of the output state.

The second is more or less the same error, seeing the outcome of a computational process as the computation itself, or conflating the process and the result. It is in fact the brain that does the computing, driven partly by the external input and partly by the rules coded as the semantic content of the informational space we call the mind (note that they are coded into the brain, as words are written on a page, but their significance lies in the informational realm). The word "space" is misleading in that it tends to imply an empty stage or arena awaiting the entry of a troupe of performers before there is any activity. However....

Definition 4.2. There is no informational space until the content is generated; as the content flickers into existence by virtue of the neuronal switching activity, it constitutes and defines a protean and ephemeral non-physical "space."

Nonetheless, there is more to accepting Rescorla's challenge to define what constitutes a "relevant sense" of computation. In one sense, the point is otiose: if it works, it's obviously relevant but, at this stage, his question can't be answered as we don't have the technology to begin to unravel the codes by which the brain computes.

The third task is of more interest. How does the concept of the brain as a computing machine relate to its neurophysiology? The answer is that it fits very well but it is important not to blur the levels of description. We can talk of the heart as a myocardium and we can talk of it as a pump. Obviously, they are closely related but they are actually different discourses, different levels of explanation of the same phenomenon. The physical heart has a structure as a bag of highly conductive muscle, which subserves its function, where the function of pumping is directly and causally-related to its structure. If we had a sufficiently developed mathematics, we could write the formulae for the heart, from its most basic structure, all the way through to its consumption of energy in pushing blood around the body.

This also applies to the standard physical description of the brain from the point of view of its anatomy, physiology and biochemistry, ranging from the level of the unaided eye down to its molecular structure. This posits the brain as a physical (extended, located) *thing* with a very wide range of physical properties.

But it is also a machine, it acquits a function, it has a performance deriving from the fundamental action of neurons, which is to conduct potential changes rapidly along their axons in such a way as to leave no trace of their passage. *But*: unlike the myocardium, neuronal action potentials have a dual role. On the one hand, they simply discharge and recover, which is pretty but uninteresting. On the other, they convey something above and beyond their "mere firing." Suitably configured, neuronal action potentials can constitute "...an *abstraction* or *representation* of physical reality..." which is the cerebral equivalent of the myocardium's function as a pump.

Finally, how does computational description relate to "...intensional description (which cites representational properties of mental states)"? Intensionality is the "aboutness" or directed content of a mental state. A mental state is *always* about something; even if it's about the idea of nothingness, it's still about something. The concept corresponds closely with Descartes' notion that if I can ask "Do I exist?" then, manifestly, I do. If I think, it's *about* something, just because that is the point of differentiation between information and noise, i.e. its intentionality or "aboutness" inheres in the definition:

Definition 4.3. There is no such thing as information devoid of content because, as an analytic truth, information just is content. Information is a representation of a state of affairs, i.e. it is necessarily a representation of some construct or other.

In other words, there cannot be a representation which is also not a representation (this was actually the first theorem that Boole proved with his new algebra of logic). Thus, the computational description is the vehicle of the intensional description, its functional complement, and there is no conflict.

4.9 The many uses of the word 'property'

Before we finish the definitions, another apology: we need to look at the concept of properties, which plagues all discussion of computational models. Rather than get lost in an interminable review, I submit that the usual use of the term *property* is completely inadequate to the tasks set for it. For example, you can find philosophers who say that bricks have the property of mass; that priests have the property of declaring a man to be a husband; that Queen Elizabeth has the property of making people bow; that paper has the property of burning; a sign has the property of making you stop; comedians have the property of making people laugh; gold has the property of value; grass has the property of being green; frogs have the property of causing fear in some people; cars have the property of transport; debates have the property of inducing boredom, and so on.

I find these disputes go nowhere because these examples involve many different senses or uses of the word. Most of the arguments could be resolved if we separate these various senses. In the remainder of this book, I will use at least the following terms to distinguish the different meanings which have attached to the word 'property':

Property: a tangible, measurable feature of an actual physical object, such as mass, height, temperature, location, velocity, pH, etc., by which we can distinguish it in the material universe. Properties are constant: they can be neither created, eliminated nor transformed but are fixed by the nature of the entity at the instant of measurement. While we may label properties in distinctive ways at our convenience, e.g. giving the wavelength of reflected light a particular name (light reflected from grass has a wavelength of 560–520 nm, which, by way of shorthand, we call *Grün*. Sorry, that's สีเขียว), the actual property involved is a physical measure which would be the same whether humans were watching it or not.

Power: A potential of an object to act in a particular way upon its surroundings, such as a rock has the power to smash glass, a cat has the power to kill a mouse, sunlight has the power of making plants grow or pale skin redden. This is wholly a physical interaction of matter and energy. It has nothing to do with what people believe or intend.

Properties and powers inhere in the object itself as it exists in the universe, and do so regardless of whether it is observed or not. Even though we have our units to measure them, these features are independent of human assessment.

Process: Any complex matter-energy transition driven by the properties and powers of a body in the physical universe, such as seeds germinating; trucks transporting goods; wounds healing; or a machine making sausages. Note two other uses of this word, such as the process of investigation (e.g. of a crime by a detective), of passing a law in Parliament, or of deciding whether a person needs an operation. The second is more contentious, as in a process of computation by a digital computer, or a process of analysis by an automated machine, such as in a biochemistry laboratory. Strictly, these are performances but by common consent, they are almost always known as processes, but be aware that the process of manufacturing sugar is conceptually of a different order from the process of determining its retail price.

Performance: Any optional action by a real entity, such as a bird doing a courtship dance; a dog chasing a cat; a football match; a speech in Parliament; people bowing to the Queen; washing the dishes; telling jokes; stitching a wound; growing food; conducting a marriage ceremony, and so on.

The remaining terms rely on a human observer to make an assessment, i.e. they are something the observer judges or concludes about an object or state of affairs. They are wholly mental constructs that do not exist until a human decides they do.

Relation: A descriptor applied to two constructs (objects, properties, powers, processes, situations etc) showing how they interact or stand in causative sequence. We need to distinguish clearly between the relationship of, say, two rocks, and the relationship of two hostile nations.

Perception: A private event occurring in inner subjective space which relates either to the external, public world (sounds, shapes, colors, odors, etc) or to the subject's personal state (pains, emotions, memories, etc). The color of gold is wholly our perception, not a property of the metal. Note that our perceptions change depending on other factors such as ambient light, even though the property (reflected light at a particular wavelength) hasn't changed. Obviously, there is some overlap between perceptions and....

Attribute: A descriptor applied by a person to an object or situation to indicate a judgement, such as the value of gold, the quality of mercy, the dearth of talent, the desirability of peace, etc. These exist only in the estimation of a human observer and have no equivalent in the natural world.

Role: A socially-determined or ordained sequence of behaviours which a person assumes or discards, depending on the rules. The Queen's role is to appoint people knights of the realm, and to look gracious while people bow; a policeman's role is to arrest robbers; a surgeon's is to perform operations; a cook's is to prepare meals and a farmer's is to grow the food. A football player's role is to kick the ball; the spectator's is to wear a silly hat and to cheer or boo according to the rules for spectators, etc. We don't say the dog's role is to chase cats as it is called instinct but a guard dog's role is to bark and growl savagely.

4.10 Information and dualism.

The concept of information is a *sine qua non* of a dualist model of mind, yet it is notoriously difficult to define. We arrived at a working definition, and used it as the basis for a computational model of how the dualist mind does its job. With this definition, some of the many problems of computational models appear to resolve. Of course, computational models just are dualist, which perhaps explains some of the hostility they attract. Another source of hostility is people who believe the human mind is so complex that we can never grasp it, perhaps because we just aren't smart enough. Granted they may find fault with this computational model but that, of course, is their role.

Finally, we clarified the term 'property' to separate physical constructs from mental attributes. This is a dualist universe: the properties of a rock are not also properties of a mental image of a rock. Rocks are heavy, but ideas about rocks aren't even weightless as they belong to a world in which the concept of weight has no meaning. The trouble is, we are so accustomed to the process of thinking that we don't even see it as astounding. In the next chapter, we will look at the processes by which immaterial thought arises from mere lumps of pink stuff, or the concept of emergence.

References

[1] Floridi L (2005). Is Semantic Information Meaningful Data? *Philosophy and Phenomenological Research* 70:(2): 351–371.
[2] Floridi L (2010). *Information: A very short introduction.* Oxford: University Press.
[3] Floridi L (2011). *The philosophy of information.* Oxford: University Press.
[4] Losee RM (1997). A discipline-independent definition of information. *Journal of the American Society for Information Science* 48(3): 254–269.

[5] Dretske FI (1983). Precis of 'Knowledge & the flow of information.' *Behavioral and Brain Sciences* 6: 55–90.

[6] Shannon CE (1948) A Mathematical Theory of Communication. *Bell System Technical Journal* 27: 379–423, 623–656 (July, October).

[7] Lenski W (2010). Information: A conceptual investigation. *Information* 1:74–118. doi:10.3390/info1020074

[8] Seising R (2010). Cybernetics, system(s) theory, information theory and Fuzzy Sets and Systems in the 1950s and 1960s. *Information Sciences* 180: 4459–4476. doi:10.1016/j.ins.2010.08.001

[9] Guizzo EM (2003) *The essential message: Claude Shannon and the making of information theory*. Unpublished masters thesis, MIT. MIT Libraries; accessed October 5th 2014.

[10] Thagard P (2008). Mental illness from the perspective of theoretical neuroscience. *Perspectives in biology and medicine* 51: 335–352.

[11] Wiener N (1948, 1965). *Cybernetics, or contol and communication in the animal and the machine*. Cambridge, MA: MIT Press.

[12] Chalmers DJ (2010). A computational foundation for the study of cognition. *Journal of Consciousness Studies* 17: 7–65.

[13] Rescorla M (2015) The Computational Theory of Mind. Stanford Encyclopaedia of Philosophy. At: https://plato.stanford.edu/entries/computational-mind/

5 The Natural Phenomenon of Emergence

Any reductionist program has to be based on an analysis of what is to be reduced... It is useless to base the defence of materialism on any analysis of mental phenomena that fails to deal explicitly with their subjective character... Without some idea, therefore, of what the subjective character of experience is, we cannot know what is required of a physicalist theory.

Thomas Nagel (b. 1937), from *What is it like to be a bat?* 1974.

5.1 Defining emergence

Emergence is the concept that unexpected novelty can arise just because the whole is more than the sum of its parts. Intuitively, most of us have no particular difficulty with it but pinning it down to some sort of formal description is notoriously difficult. There are various definitions around, for example:

An emergent phenomenon displays causal powers not displayed by any of its parts; or,

An emergent property of an entity is a novel property not displayed by, contained in or implied by any of its constituents in isolation.

Moreover, the concept of emergence is highly contentious, not least because admitting the phenomenon of emergence seems to allow all sorts of unwanted matters. For example, working within a materialist framework, a theorist would want to exclude such things as telekinesis, out-of-body experiences, prescience and so on. However, if she allows emergence, she really can't object when somebody says, "Aha, but your science doesn't exclude emergence, and these are emergent phenomena, so you must accept them." People therefore tend to avoid the notion of emergence because it may open the door to magic. Avoiding the taint of magic was a major factor in the twentieth century program of trying to write mind out of science.

Historically, the term emergence dates from the philosopher George Lewes (1817–1878) who described two sorts of novel properties, resultant and emergent (1875). Resultant properties are what we get when we mix things or add

DOI: 10.4324/9781003183792-5

them together: the weight of a box of rocks is the combined weight of all the rocks plus the box. This can be predicted from weighing them individually. An emergent property could not be predicted, and he mostly related it to life forms. A century and a half ago, the battle between physicalists and vitalists was still being fought. Physicalists claimed that all properties and behaviours of living organisms can be fully explained by reference to the properties of the chemical constituents of each organism. Not so, replied the vitalists, that will never be enough. There has to be an extra factor - vital fluid, entelechy, spirit, call it what you will – but it is not of the material universe, so a physical investigation of a living organism will always be incomplete. Emergentists found a niche in between these extremes. Their view was that physical investigation will not explain all of life but the novel properties are natural, not supernatural, and, even if we can't predict them beforehand, we can probably understand them after the event. However, as they often didn't add, it was also unlikely that ordinary reductive biology would explain them because taking an organism apart destroys the emergent properties we are trying to understand.

Starting with Friedrich Wöhler's (1800–1882) synthesis of urea in 1828, the processes of "life" were gradually explained in terms of biochemistry, molecular physiology and genetics, meaning the physicalists ultimately won and vitalism faded away. Insofar as orthodox psychiatry claims that all mental disorder will be fully explained by reference to the brain's chemistry, it resides firmly within the physicalist camp. In a fully reductionist or physicalist psychiatry, there is no room and no need for "mind." Modern physicalists, such as the neurophysiologist Eric Kandel (b. 1929) [1] and the philosopher Paul Thagard (b. 1950) [2], have loudly proclaimed that their programs will eventually triumph via some Grand Theory of Everything. They were not mindful of the work of theoretical physicist, Phillip Anderson (1923–2020) who, in a classic paper published in 1972, warned against what he called the reductionist approach, characterised thus:

> The workings of our minds and bodies, and of all the animate or inanimate matter of which we have any detailed knowledge, are assumed to be controlled by the same set of fundamental laws, which except under certain extreme conditions, we feel we know pretty well... if everything obeys the same fundamental laws, then the only scientists who are studying anything really fundamental are those who are working on those laws [3].

He mounted a clear case against what would now be called *physicalism*, showing how at each stage of complexity, new laws and generalisations are required to account for the observable phenomena:

> At each stage (of complexity), entirely new laws, concepts, and generalizations are necessary, requiring inspiration and creativity to just as great a degree as in the previous one. Psychology is not applied biology, nor is biology applied chemistry (p393)

Since then, the information revolution has dealt a severe blow to physicalist ambitions. Information is about symbols: symbols can be causally effective and yet they are not reducible to their physical substrate. Symbols "emerge" from the physical machine but are not part of the machine, nor are they specific to just that machine. For reductionists, they are ontological loose threads, the point at which reductionism fails just because the whole purpose of reductionism is to get rid of all the "loose threads" purists saw in dualism (the major loose thread in any dualist theory is interaction of body and mind, which we will come to).

5.2 Characteristics of emergence

Philosopher Paul Humphreys (b. 1950) [4] nominated six characteristics of emergence:

1   *Novelty:* "A previously uninstantiated property[1] comes to have an instance."
2   *Qualitative difference:* "Emergent properties (are) qualitatively different from the properties from which they emerge."
3   *Absence at lower levels:* "An emergent property is one that could not be possessed at a lower level – it is logically or nomologically impossible for this to occur."
4   *Law difference:* "Different laws apply to emergent features than to the features from which they emerge."
5   *Interactivity:* "Emergent properties... result from an essential interaction between their constituent properties."
6   *Holism:* "Emergent properties are holistic in the sense of being properties of the entire system rather than local properties of its constituents."

More recently, and after detailed explication, Humphreys has proposed that four criteria capture the essence of emergentism: emergence is relational (i.e. emergent entities must result from something else); novelty, autonomy and holism [5]. A lot of his argument relies on extensive philosophical knowledge and is not immediately accessible to people trained in biology so I will follow his earlier approach.

David Chalmers [6] sees two forms of emergence, strong and weak. Strong emergence means that the truths or properties of a higher-order entity are not predictable or deducible in principle from the truths or properties of the lower-order entities of which it is composed. This tends to be the way it is used in philosophy, even though Humphreys uses it differently:

> ...an entity... is strongly emergent only if it has the ability to causally influence entities at a lower level by means of features that belong to the

---

1   Note that he tends to conflate the different uses of the term 'properties' that were separated at the end of Chapter 4.

emergent entity but that are not found in structured aggregates of lower level entities... it is widely held that strong emergence is either an incoherent or an unscientific position [6, p. 50].[2]

In this section, I will rely on Chalmers' usage but, as Humphreys noted, it is an uncomfortable concept because it can mean that, even with the wisdom of hindsight, we may not be able to account for the novel features. In this sense, it isn't clear how it differs from the idea of "mysterianism," the concept that we can never understand fully how mind arises from brain, when Chalmers clearly does want to understand it. Weak emergence says that while the properties of the higher-order entity may be unexpected, we can readily account for them in retrospect. This tends to be the way the word emergence is used in science because it precludes unexplained entities: in science, we have to be able to account for every observation. Anything we can't explain may be put aside briefly but it can't be ignored indefinitely.

Chalmers asked:

> ...are there strongly emergent phenomena?...yes. I think there is exactly one clear case of a strongly emergent phenomenon, and that is the phenomenon of consciousness.

At first, this looks as though he is begging the question but he is actually saying: "If there are any strongly emergent phenomena, then I am nominating conscious experience as the most likely, if not the only, candidate." That's a legitimate move as it charts a research program. Conscious experience, he says, is not predictable from physical principles or properties prior to the event, nor deducible after the event, because it is not a product of physical properties or principles. It supervenes upon the brain's organisation by psychophysical laws that we can eventually understand, even though he makes no suggestion as to what these might be. This is a bit risky; it smacks of *deus ex machina*. Earlier, I proposed that Chalmers' "psychophysical laws" governing the emergence of mind may just be George Boole's "Laws of Thought," or derive directly from them. Boole's "Laws" are the most basic requirements for the emergence of higher order mental properties, even if they aren't sufficient.

5.3 Emergence and computational capacity of brain

In the terms defined by George Boole, the emergence of mind is explicable as a product of the brain's computational capacity. As such, it depends utterly on the organisational principles or algorithms that govern the data processing (programs, if you wish). At no point, prior to or after the event of any informational state, is there anything inherent in the physical properties of the material universe

---

2 Humphreys would characterise the model being developed here as strong transformational ontological emergence [5, Chap. 2].

that would allow us to explain the informational state in material terms, just because an informational state does not arise from, is not governed by, and does not reduce to the laws of the material universe. While an informational state is permitted by the laws of the physical universe, it is truly emergent but it does not thereby breach the laws of thermodynamics; they are beside the point, as Shannon noted ("These semantic aspects of communication are irrelevant to the engineering problem"). That is, there is nothing about electrons that determines your sense of humour or your knowledge of the traffic laws. Similarly, while molecules are devoid of morality, the idea of an immoral molecule is a category error (Gilbert Ryle: properties or entities belonging to one category are presented as though they belong to another category [7]). If our fragile morality is not inscribed on our molecules, whence does it derive? By exclusion, it can only flow from our molecules doing whatever molecules do once they are cast in the form of logic gates. That is the definition of performance, and morality is a performance, not a property or power. Performances are learned, not innate.

Only an entity with an emergent informational state or mind can recognise such states in other entities, but not all such informational states have sufficient computational power to grasp the concepts that brought them into being.

In the same vein, I do not believe that the contents of the Bible (or any other book) are determined by the physical properties of the paper on which it is printed. Nor were they determined by the purely physical properties of the molecules of the brains of the prophets, or the scribes or anybody. As the table game Scrabble shows, mere matter does not determine informational content, it's what you do with it that counts. By acting as its mechanism, physical matter can carry informational content, but that's of entirely a different order. This also applies to the rules of cricket, of etiquette, of the use of the subjunctive in French, the treaties on the rights of the mentally ill, the choice of colours on national flags, and so on. There is nothing in the spin of the electron, the mass of a neutron or the charge of a proton that determines these questions, because they do not belong to the material universe. Anybody who claims otherwise is making an unsubstantiated (ideological) claim, one which constitutes a category error.

That, however, is only half the case. The other half is that, armed with my own informational state, meaning my mind, I can fully comprehend the generic case for informational states as the products of certain sorts of coordinated switching in suitable machines. In this approach, there is no such thing as strong emergence as we can always understand it in these (informational) terms. Because we ourselves have informational processing capacities, we can readily tell whether another machine or organism will also have them, although we cannot predict what it will be like to be one of those entities. Perhaps we never will, as it would depend on knowing the codes in which the information is expressed. But I now believe it is only a matter of time before we can program digital computers to develop a form of experience not substantially different from our own. Whether we should do this, or whether anthropogenic climate change will overtake us first, are entirely different questions.

Let's return to Humphreys' principles and see whether the concept of an emergent mind satisfies them.

1   *Novelty:* Yes, I believe there was a time on the planet Earth when there was nothing that could in any sense have possessed mental properties, e.g. while the planet was still a pile of molten rock. At one stage, there were no mental properties but now there are.

2   *Qualitative difference:* That's easy, minds have properties, powers and performances that bricks and brains don't.

3   *Absence at lower levels:* A healthy, intact brain has powers that a single neuron, or the pituitary, or the cerebellum, do not.

4   *Law difference:* Absolutely. The law of gravity applies to neurons but not to daydreams.

5   *Interactivity:* What we call 'mind' is the result of the interaction of a very large number of highly specialised *biological* elements (neurons, assembled in the form of a healthy brain) operating within very tightly specified physical parameters. If those elements are isolated so they can no longer interact, then the mental properties cease to be. Similarly, if the system ventures outside its physiological limits, mental function degrades, then halts.

6   *Holism:* True, half a brain just won't do.

Conscious experience *emerges* by virtue of subtle and sophisticated, recursive processing of data within the brain's dedicated switching mechanisms. It is an emergent product of the material realm but is not thereby material in its own right. Mind is irreducibly *sui generis,* a thing unto itself.

5.4 On free will

The question of whether we have the capacity to control our actions is ancient – and vexatious. The idea of free will is that, regardless of how I acted one minute ago, I could have acted differently. The principle behind freedom of will is that all events have prior causes, and that we had control over these prior causes. Extreme determinists take the view that we don't have this option, that all our actions (including thinking we have freedom of choice) are predetermined by one means or another, all of which lie outside our control. Indeed, they say, the universal sense that we have the freedom to choose and act differently, that there are decision points, is an illusion (although I have never heard any reductionist explain why the illusion exists, since it would have no survival value). Benedict Spinoza (1632–77) put it succinctly:

> There is no such thing as Freewill. The mind is induced to wish this or that by some cause, and that cause is determined by another cause, and so on back to infinity.

However, this implies that, in the absolute beginning, *either* all events had the same cause, or the universe sprang into being with a myriad causes already in place, which isn't much help. In the case of physicalism, which says that the properties of mind are reducible to and fully explained as a matter of the properties of the physical structure of the brain, it is hard to maintain a case for free will. In this view, the final cause for any mental event is a physical event; therefore, all mental events should ultimately be governed by the laws of the physical universe. *Prima facie,* for anybody who accepts biological reductionism, this would be a compelling argument against the notion of freedom of choice: how can molecules control themselves? Molecules are strictly governed by the laws of physics so, in the physicalist view, it would follow that a full understanding of an individual's brain would tell us exactly what she will do at all stages of her life.

Opposing this is the humanist view, which argues that the claim that we don't have self-control is not just wrong, but is a brutal negation of everything that society stands for. The concept of morality, inherent in all societies and all religions as far back as we know, depends absolutely on the notion that we are responsible for what we do. Our system of laws presupposes that a person has the ability and the duty to make rational decisions; all things being equal, when people break the law, they could have done otherwise and must be held liable. We have an elaborate system of statutes and case law to govern those examples when we feel that a person has acted illegally but without full self-control, and psychiatry operates at least partly within this field. It would be self-contradictory for a psychiatrist to say that a mentally-disordered person has a biological disease of the brain over which he has no control, but is also responsible in law for all his actions.

Opposing this, the dualist model says that the prior cause of a mental event consists of other mental events, without limit. An extreme rationalist view, such as that espoused by Thomas Szasz, (1920–2012) argues that everything we do is the outcome of rational choices, even to the extent of choosing to be "mentally ill." Even though Szasz inspires ferocious support among his followers, I believe his concepts are incoherent [8]. Freudian psychology takes the view that we aren't as rational as we like to think, that a very large chunk of our behaviour is governed by hidden mental events of a primitive nature over which we have little or no control. However, psychoanalysis says that we can gain control over them and behave more rationally.

Regardless, we do in fact have free will because, prior to or even in the midst of an action, we can always review our mental "prior causes" and revise them to give a more appropriate outcome. Through our capacity to represent states of affairs in a symbolic calculus, we can look ahead, we can predict where our actions are heading and change them, before they happen. That's what information processors do; that's why they're information processors and why they dominate, say, plants, which can't model the future. That's the advantage of being an information processor: we can change our own settings, as it were, at no cost to the matter-energy balance of the universe. The biocognitive model accepts that humans have a considerable degree of freedom of choice, although we are not always as rational as we like to think. If I am constrained always to act according to some imposed standard of rationality, then I don't have freedom of choice, I am not free. Rationality Police and Moral Police wear the same uniform, only their badges are different.

To summarise, we distinguish between, on the one hand, resultant properties and powers and, on the other, emergent performances. An emergent phenomenon is one that shows novel performances that cannot be predicted from knowledge of the properties and powers of its constituent elements. For example, the liquidity of water at 10C and normal pressure, gravity etc. are *necessary* and, therefore, given a sufficient knowledge of physics, predictable before the event and explicable after. On the other hand, the capacity of a switching system to generate an informational state is not a necessary performance. While it is explicable after the event, it is unpredictable beforehand. In particular, the informational content is infinite and is therefore always unpredictable. After the event, it can be described ("Oh, well, that's just what it says") but it cannot be explained other than in informational terms.

The mind is a bundle of emergent performances, one of which is recursion, meaning self-control or self-direction. That is, emergence leads to free will whereas resultant properties don't. I can decide to move out of the hot sun or stay in it, as the fancy takes me, whereas a tree can't.

References

[1] Kandel ER (2005). *Psychiatry, psychoanalysis and the new biology of mind.* Washington, DC: American Psychiatric Publishing.
[2] Thagard PR (2008). Mental Illness from the Perspective of Theoretical Neuroscience. *Perspect Biol Med* 51 (3): 335–352.
[3] Anderson PW (1972). More is different: broken symmetry and the nature of the heirarchical structure of science. *Science.* 177 (4047): 393–396.
[4] Humphreys P (1997). Emergence, not Supervenience. *Philosophy of Science.* 64: S337–S345.
[5] Humphreys P (2016). *Emergence: a philosophical account.* New York: Oxford UP.
[6] Chalmers DJ (2006). Strong and Weak Emergence. In Clayton P, Davies P, (eds.) *The Re-emergence of Emergence.* Oxford: University Press.
[7] Ryle G (1949). *The Concept of Mind.* London: Hutchinson.
[8] McLaren N (2012). Critical review of Thomas Szasz. Chapters 12, 13 in *The Mind-Body Problem Explained: The Biocognitive Model for Psychiatry.* Ann Arbor, MI: Future Psychiatry Press

Part II
Implementation

6 Information and the brain

I remember at an early period of my own life showing to a man of high reputation as a teacher some matters which I happened to have observed. And I was very much struck and grieved to find that, while all the facts lay equally clear before him, only those that squared with his previous theories seemed to affect his organs of vision.

Joseph Lister, 1st Baron (1827–1912)

The reasonable man adapts himself to the world. The unreasonable man persists in trying to adapt the world to himself. All progress, therefore, depends on the unreasonable man.

George Bernard Shaw (1856–1950)
Maxims for Revolutionists No. 124

An idea that is not dangerous is unworthy of being called an idea at all.

Oscar Wilde (1854–1900).

6.1 The mind as an informational space.

So far, we have spoken of mind as an informational space in the most general, theoretical terms. All good, you say, I accept the possibility that the brain may have that sort of capacity but two questions arise. Firstly, is it true that the brain is capable of supporting that sort of model, and secondly, as a matter of empirical fact, does it do so? In Sects. 3.3 – 3.4, we briefly sketched some of the basic considerations in answering these questions. In this chapter, we will look in more detail at the brain as we understand it today. Bear in mind that the human central nervous system is the most complex thing in the known universe, so complex that some people say we can never understand it. Be that as it may, the field of neurophysiology is developing very rapidly, even though some of today's hot research programs will surely turn out to be dead-ends.

Sect. 3.4 sets out the case for the human brain being a very high-powered digital data processor, with something of the order of 120trillion (10^{12}) logic gates available just for executive functions. Of course, all the logic gates in the universe aren't much help without the requisite software to operate them but we

DOI: 10.4324/9781003183792-6

know nothing about that aspect of brain function. Indeed, we may never know because every attempt to study the problem could result in the death of the subject. On the other hand, we probably don't need to know that sort of detail because a much coarser level will tell us enough to solve human problems.

Does that sound familiar? As a historical point, there has already been one attempt to understand human behaviour at a coarse level, in fact, at the coarsest possible level. Behaviorism tried to write the mind out of the equation. Forget what goes on inside the head, excited psychologists shouted, all that counts is the relationship between stimulus and response. That failed, of course: it isn't possible to write the mind out of the equation. You may think you've done it but all you've done is shift the intelligence that needs to be explained from one point to another. One of the most determined behaviorists of all, Burrhus F Skinner (1904–1990) invented a box to find the formulae governing stimulus and response. It was designed to show that the behaviour of animals such as pigeons and rats could be analysed in S-R terms to the point where it became possible to "predict and control" the animal's future behavior. The mechanism of the Skinner Box restricted the subject animal to either-or responses to any stimulus.

Using this method, Skinner showed (at least to his satisfaction) that complex behaviour could be reduced to very simple equations. What he didn't realise was that these animals, and in fact all animals, actually live in much richer and more complex environments than in his laboratory. He removed the role of intelligence in governing behaviour and hid it in the environment: it took a lot of intelligence to decide that there is no such thing as a mind (he was never clear on this point) and to devise his box and the experimental schedules he used. Yes, we can make pigeons look dumb; we can actually do that to humans, too, by placing them in a restricted environment such as a prison or a mental hospital, but it takes a lot of intellect to do it and it doesn't prove the point. In fact, all Skinner did was invent a new language to *describe* behaviour; he didn't explain it at all [1].

We don't want to repeat that mistake so we will work at the level of natural languages on the assumption that, ultimately, they are based in the dual-valued logic developed by George Boole, and that this logic accurately reflects the *functional architecture* of the brain's neurons.

6.2 Executive functions: the easy problem

Basic experiment: a person is seated in a comfortable chair looking at a screen. His instructions are simple: "If you see a patch of colour that is not the colour of blood or the colour of grass, press the pedal under your non-dominant foot." Shortly, a patch of blue appears on the screen. He presses his right foot on a pedal, ending the experiment. "Oh," says the technician, "you're left-handed, are you?" The subject nods agreement and leaves the room.

There are two features of this little experiment to explain, one summarised by Chalmers' "easy problem of consciousness" and the other the hard problem. We will start with the easy one, the question of deciding what to do, or executive function. Beginning at the level of the eye, light from the screen strikes the colour receptors in the retina, provoking a burst of nerve impulses in the optic nerve that travel toward the brain (the afferent flow). This first or transduction step is very important: exteroceptors are either nerve endings themselves or are cells activated by specific energy inputs which act directly on neurons, causing them to discharge. It is by this means that information from the external world is received and translated into nerve impulses, the basic "language" of the brain. Until this takes place, nothing happens in the brain. During neurosurgery on an alert patient, the surgeon can shine a torch on the subject's brain but its owner will not perceive anything just because the cerebral cortex is incapable of converting light energy into nerve impulses. That can only take place in specialised receptor cells in the retina, just as sound is converted into nerve impulses by specialised receptor cells in the organ of Corti in the inner ear. The latter are mechanoreceptors, triggered by physical movement, whereas the retinal cells are photoreceptors only. If, however, the cortex is stimulated by electricity, the subject will experience something, depending on the area stimulated, because electric currents can activate neurons.

On the receptor or afferent side of the brain, the first step of the junction between the world and the mind is a receptor neuron which has the unique property of converting physical energy to nerve impulses.

The optic nerve input is not colour itself, it is a highly derivative representation of a specific state of affairs, being patterns of different wavelengths of light in the external world. Presumably, the pattern evoked today by the colour blue will be the same as blue evokes tomorrow, but that's not important. The afferent flow is further processed in the thalamus, at the lateral geniculate nucleus, composed of nerve cell bodies responsible for the visual functions of determining range and velocity of an object (in our experiment, these parameters were eliminated). Their axons then project via the optic radiation to the primary visual cortex in the occipital region of the brain.

By this stage, we can differentiate two further types of neuronal function, the conduit or transmission function, and the processing or sorting function. Transduction, transmission and processing; there is one further function we will come to later.

As much (or as little) as we now know about the cerebral cortex, it remains a mystery how it does its job. The incoming data flow is processed and reprocessed in cascades of precisely-organised neurons, with two outcomes, as this experiment shows. The more immediate is the ineffable experience of seeing something blue, but almost simultaneously, there is a decision at the level of communicable knowledge, *blue*. Because we're dealing with the easy problem first, we'll focus on the second response. Neurons stimulated by a particular wavelength of light (in this case, between about 450–490nm) sent signals to the cortex where they interacted with signals previously coded and stored in memory, summarised as:

$$(\neg R \wedge \neg G) \rightarrow R \text{ foot.}$$

The subject already knows that *Not the colour of blood* = Not red, *Not grass* = Not green, and *Non-dominant foot* = Right foot. Here we have Boole's rules of thought in action, the reduction of a complex instruction to a series of elementary steps in a dual-valued calculus that imply no mystery on behalf of the organ implementing them.

The critical point is that all of this takes place at the level of neuronal impulses being shunted through a series of logic gates coded into the walls of the receiving neurons, but the physical mechanism of this calculation, and its informational content, are always ontologically distinct and must not be conflated. At no point in its journey from retina to calf muscles does the nature of the physical mechanism subserving the information flow change: it is wholly a matter of observable nerve impulses. While the physical mechanism remains constant, at some point in the cerebral cortex, the *significance* of the impulses changes. Before reaching the occipital cortex, it is mainly a matter of raw data pulsing through the transmission section of the pathway (the afferent axons) but this changes in the brain proper. Here, data flows through cascades of neurons where it can interact with instructions stored in memory. In this model, reversible changes to functional logic gates built into the neuronal wall constitute the physical basis of memory. A new memory is simply a matter of resetting the particular logic gates involved in the decision.

It should be apparent that all of this takes place at a level outside "consciousness," meaning at a level we can't access. We can access the various inputs ("Why did you press with your right foot?" "Because you said non-dominant, and I'm left-handed") and we are apprised of the output, but the actual process or mechanism of reaching a decision is forever hidden from us. And probably with good reason: it would simply distract from the real problem of evading a large and hungry carnivore.

6.3 Executive functions: the hard problem

This is a solution to the easy bit of the easy problem of consciousness; I am definitely not saying it is *the* solution. The hard bit of the easy problem is accounting for creativity. We can readily understand how, one pleasant summer evening, William Shakespeare decided to stop work briefly to open the door to let the cat out, but what happened when he sat down again at his table, picked up his quill and got back to work on *Hamlet?* According to Mark Forsyth (b. 1977) in his book, *The Elements of Eloquence*, he did it the same way as a sculptor carves a statue: chip by chip or, in the case of a playwright, penstroke by penstroke, word by word [2]. Shakespeare found a story he liked, roughed it out, then sat down and began to rework every sentence, every couplet, every word indeed, until he felt it would be safe to present it to the very choosy denizens of South London.

George Boole's own story illustrates the process of creativity. The quote from his widow in Sect. 2.2 describes how, at the age of seventeen, he had a "flash of psychological insight" into how we acquire knowledge. But this didn't come out of the blue to a youth who was more interested in girls and fishing than in matters of mentation. It happened because he had been engrossed in the question at about the same time as he had been studying logic and algebra. For a large part of each day, he tossed the ideas around in his head, worrying them, fitting them this way and that until he chanced upon the right formula. Suddenly, what people thought were unrelated ideas clicked together and he saw the deeper connections. Thereafter, he devoted decades of work to turn the bare bones of his insight into theorems of logic.

There is nothing magic about this. In the first place, how does any answer suggest itself? Turing outlined the processes involved, as described in Sect. 2.4:

> Any question that a human can ask... can be broken down into a series of sub-questions. These can be further broken down, again and again until all that is left is a series of questions that are so simple that a dumb machine can answer them by, for example, choosing which is the larger of two numbers.

This is computed for us, in that we aren't aware of and can't access the mechanisms involved. The "flash of insight," which we have all experienced at some stage, is a dumb, mechanical process, a matter of chance, of a nugget flashing among the dross. Every idea on how to solve a problem is computed for us, but very often, it's wrong. How many times a day do we think: "Aha, I know the answer, I'll... No, that wouldn't work"? People who are satisfied with the status quo don't develop new ideas just because they see no need for change, they don't toss ideas around in their heads, they don't actively search for nuggets. Nuggets are found by people working hard, worrying a problem, most often in isolation, while everybody else is enjoying a day at the beach or getting over a hangover. GB Shaw summarised it well in the opening quote to this chapter.

We can reduce a large part of the process of creating novelty to one simple rule: Find fault. Use your intellect to find fault in an idea by comparing what you see with whatever your concepts of the world tell you ought to be. If you have the feeling that something's not quite right, even though everybody else accepts it as good enough, believe that you're right and don't give up just because other people laugh. As Thomas Edison said, genius is 1% inspiration and 99% perspiration, so tear down the ideas of the great and self-satisfied, find their weaknesses and don't stop until something better emerges. Never be satisfied, especially with your own work. Bold new ideas or inventions no more emerge intact from the inner darkness than, say, the sculptures of Mt Rushmore emerged from the South Dakota ranges one Saturday afternoon. A lot of work went into them, just as a lot of work went into Boole's Laws of Thought.

So what is the nature of the "nugget," the kernel of an idea that can be shaped into something worthwhile? There is no firm answer to that yet, because we would have to know the codes by which the brain operates. It depends on how we code ideas but the basic mechanism of solving problems is the same, regardless of how big or small. The psychologist Jean Piaget showed how our capacity to reason develops from concrete operations to abstract operations, and that is very much a process of building exponentially on acquired skills. Which monkeys do quite well.

6.4 The hard problem of consciousness

It would be nice to say there is an easy bit to start the process but if there is, I haven't heard of it. The subject matter of the hard problem of consciousness is the concept of experiencing something (qualia if you wish, sensations if you don't), such that being awake and aware is something that being in a deep sleep is not. Despite the protestations of behaviorists and physicalist philosophers, pain, fear, misery, hunger, dreams and all other emotions and experiences are real. They are just not of the realm that we ordinarily call "real." That is, there are two classes of real matters, public and private, neither of which can be gainsaid. Normally, we divide the real private matters into emotions and sensations but I propose that the mechanism underlying the two groups is essentially the same. As with decision-making, the mechanism of the experience is a matter of data processing, the manipulation of a representation of the outside world by a prodigiously powerful data-processing device (the brain), according to principles acquired during early development.

Honed by hundreds of millions of years of evolution, the animal brain organises itself in such a way as to maximise our awareness of, and responsivity to, subtle differences in the external environment. A central part of that is the creation of a complex and unique informational space, probably by recursive processing of the data flow, to exaggerate slight changes in the energy input. Thus, red looks very different from yellow, even though there is scant difference in their wavelengths. We presume animals that developed the capacity to perceive such differences had a survival advantage over those that didn't. Yes, cats are color-blind but they are nocturnal carnivores. Their eyes are specialised for detecting movement in low light intensity, so colour vision, which requires much greater light flux, is of no use to them.

This may say *why* we see red but it doesn't answer the question of *how* we actually see red, or hear the sound of danger. Needless to say, I don't know. The mysterian would say "I told you so. We can never know, we aren't smart enough." The behaviorist would say "Stop worrying, it's a pseudo-problem." The physicalist would say "A full understanding of the brain will tell us." I believe all these responses are wrong. We can be sure that seeing red, or hearing a rustle in the grass, has something to do with digital data flows in neurons, because that's how the data is presented to the brain. Absent magic, there isn't anything else available.

Moreover, we can be sure the data flow is processed in a coherent way, that the experience depends upon the processing, that the processing is done according to acquired principles (rules) acting upon neuronal activity (the data flow) in an innate or genetically-determined physical substrate (the brain itself). We know that the phenomenon of experience has been around for a long time so it probably doesn't need much computing power, and that the product of that processing is necessarily ephemeral (because each time a neuron discharges, which it does in the order of milliseconds, it returns precisely to *status quo ante*, thereby obliterating the experience). Finally, the outcome is wholly private to the individual because there is no direct means of contact between one brain and the next. That may come, of course, but, in trying to understand the process of emergence of the experiences, the possibility doesn't concern us.

Just because they are built on the information coded in a data flow, all mental states are necessarily *about* something. Information is *always* about something, because that's what information means. If a data flow isn't *about* something, it's called noise. Somehow, the neuronal data flow generates a sense of something distinct from and in contrast to oblivion, such as during an anesthetic or the oblivion that existed before we were born. That something results from a very brief, even instantaneous, recursive manipulation of the input data flow such that, for a barely perceptible span, it acts back upon itself. It has to be brief (i.e. heavily damped), because anything else would inevitably set up an infinite circuit, which would would quickly bring the entire system to a halt.

As a crude physical analogy, imagine the streams of sparks from two fireworks passing through each other. At the instant of their intersection, they generate something that isn't true of or contained in either stream of sparks. That is, an ephemeral image emerges which, for the instant before it is obliterated, seems bigger than, but not implied by, either flow of sparks. In this example, it is perfectly feasible that the larger image would not be predicted beforehand, and not inconceivable that it could not be explained after the event, i.e. it could be chaotic, where chaos is defined as the property of a complex system whose behaviour, owing to great sensitivity to small changes in conditions, is subject to so many factors as to appear random,. Even though the latter possibility would appeal to a mysterian, I don't like it but I can't find a convincing case against it.

The standard objection to this admittedly imperfect analogy is that it needs an observer to complete the model, which immediately leads to an infinite regress. That would be true except in the single case where the created entity was its own observer, which is true of humans, except we call the process of observation conscious awareness. Once again, we can't make much progress with this until we know the brain's actual codes, which may forever be beyond us. At the same time, it's not that important to the model, because whatever the exact mechanism, it is instantiated by algorithms operating within the larger model of the mind as an informational space generated by the brain's capacity to process data. We don't need to know that level of detail to be able to understand and predict behavior.

Within the central nervous system (CNS), there are many subsystems that contribute to our capacity to survive. Apart from the physiological systems, these are end-state or independent output functions. Thus, a person with damage to the auditory cortex will function perfectly well in all other systems. Working together, held together by the cement of memory, these subsystems give an impression of a unity that is simply not based in fact. Take away all these subsystems and we aren't left with "pure consciousness," we are left with.... nothing. Oblivion. The unity of self is a phantom, a fragile illusion that splits apart under even slight pressure such as sleep deprivation, fever, chemicals and other toxic agents, concussion and, above all, fear.

6.5 Output states: the path of executive functions

As you would imagine, output states are whatever an entity achieves through its activity. The output state of a muscle is motion (and heat, H_2O and CO_2 etc); the output state of a leaf is sugars + H_2O + O_2; the output state of a car is transport + hot gases + noise, and so on. The output state of the executive or decision-making part of the brain is, of course, decisions, but they have to be effected before they can have any impression on the world. In the little experiment in Sect. 6.2, the subject was given some instructions, which he encoded in memory. Subsequently, these were used in a computation involving coded information from the visual system to send an instruction to the muscles of the calf.

Computationally, this is very simple stuff. The important point in the biocognitive model of mind is that the various items of information in the experiment came from different sources (ears, eyes, memory) and were able to interact causally just because they were implemented in the same architecture, as spike impulses in neurons. All information in the CNS is coded in this form so, potentially, all information in the CNS can interact to influence the outcome state. As mentioned previously, the mechanism of memorising instructions may be no more than a matter of resetting logic gates but that isn't important. The information interacts rapidly, the process of computation isn't accessible or reportable, but it is still under the individual's control just because each person sets his or her own rules and is therefore responsible for them. Even in the case of the many rules acquired very early in life, even preverbally, each person is fully liable for them.

If you are one of those lucky people who had a good family life, you will probably have a fairly benign set of rules about yourself, the world and your place in it. Most likely, you will believe that the world is a nice place full of interesting possibilities and, if you want or need something, all you have to do is ask, or maybe do a bit of light work, and it will drop into your lap. If you want help, you know that a quick call or two will have friends and relatives rallying around so there is never any cause for alarm. Really, the world is a fascinating place full of lovely, helpful, caring, considerate and amusing people. They're the rules your early life experiences allowed you to draw. They mesh together smoothly, with each other and with the world itself but, even with no reason to question them, they're still your rules.

On the other hand, you may have been brought into the world by a pair of drunken, brawling, dishonest misfits who didn't want you and regard you as the cause of all the trouble that has happened in their miserable lives. Given that sort of welcome, it is most likely that you will come to believe that the world is a treacherous place full of deadly traps. To make it worse, you may have believed half of the terrible things your relatives said about you. You will know that if you want or need something, you must never tell anybody otherwise they will do everything they can to make sure you don't get it. If by some chance you've managed to get something, look out because everybody is out to steal it. On the other hand, if you didn't get it, that only proves what a cruel and heartless world it is. If you want help, don't let anybody know because as soon as they realise you've hit a rough patch, they'll really put the boot in. You may have a few friends but you'll never trust them fully because they'll do the dirty on you if they can, yet having your relatives around is cause for panic. In brief, the world is a harsh, punitive place full of selfish, brutal, dishonest and otherwise terrifying people. They're the rules that, in order to survive, your early life experiences forced you to draw. As rules, they are inconsistent, they grate and jar and set you up for trouble, but trouble always comes your way, meaning nothing ever happens to give you reason to question them. They're still your rules.

We all have rules, we run our lives according to rules. If you didn't know the rules of English, you wouldn't be able to read this but how many of you can point to the most recent example of the future subjunctive tense I have used? Possibly very few, but most readers would have understood what it meant, even had it been used incorrectly. Our rules make us what we are just because they are coded into the brain and thereby govern our decisions. With our rules in place, physical energy from the external world impacts on specialised transducer cells in the sensory organs and is converted into nerve impulses. Once in the common cerebral language, rules and sensory input can interact, decisions are made and instructions are sent to the different muscle groups via the vastly complex cerebellar systems.

Mind and body have two junctions. The initial or input junction of mind and body lies on the sensory or afferent side of the CNS where information from the receptor organs is transduced before being transmitted to the computational regions of the brain. The second is on the effector or efferent side, where decisions are directed to the particular effector organs. In between the sensory input and the effector output, information from a variety of sources, cast in the common neuronal language, is integrated and an outcome determined. The second or output junction of mind and body is the point where the last computational neuron in the system acts upon the first transmission neuron leading to the effector organ.

On the effector or efferent side of the brain, the final step in the junction between the mind and the world is the motor end-plate of the spinal motor neuron, whose unique role is to convert nerve impulses to physical movement. When impulses travel down the motor nerve from the brain, they reach the motor end-plate which causes the release of a chemical, acetyl choline. This diffuses across the tiny gap between the nerve ending and the muscle cells, causing the muscle to start to depolarise. From that point, a wave of depolarisation spreads across the surface of the muscle, which leads its internal protein structure to contract. That is, the spinal motor neuron "speaks the language" of the muscle fibre. By this means, a thought such as a decision to act is conveyed from the brain to a point where it is converted into motor activity. We can legitimately say that a mechanism exists by which thoughts control behavior.

6.6 Output states: the path of physiological functions

Physiological functions follow a similar path in that there is a particular point at which nerve impulses conveying instructions from the brain are converted into secretions, which then act upon the physical body in the usual way. This takes place in *neurosecretory neurons*, many of which are located in the hypothalamus, particularly in the preoptic and suprachiasmatic regions. At its receiving or dendritic end, a neurosecretory neuron is just like any other neuron but at its distal or axonic end, it has specialised organelles which do not impinge on a further neuron. Given a particular pattern of impulses, these release specific chemicals which diffuse into the bloodstream and thence activate distal organs. It is a two-step process, of converting nerve impulses into chemicals (releasing factors), which then stimulate their target organ into releasing a further chemical (hormone). Thus, we can legitimately say that thoughts control aspects of bodily physiology, which would not have surprised the ancient Greeks, or Indians, or most other races. It is only shocking in the context of Western society's "....overwhelmingly physicalist or materialist intellectual culture...." (Daniel Stoljar, [3,4]).

In humans, one hormone in particular is directly affected by the mental state, testosterone. This hormone, which is very widespread in nature, has a complex physiology with two main effects. The first is the well-known androgenising effect, meaning preparing the male body for reproduction. The second is anabolic, building muscle bulk, stimulating bone growth and density and, importantly, inducing a feeling of strength and confidence. However, a crucial role of this hormone is often overlooked, and it is not restricted to humans, even though it is very obvious in our species. This is known as the *Challenge Hypothesis*, the notion that in order to meet a challenge, the animal must produce a burst of testosterone to be physically and mentally prepared for the contest. This has been described in detail in Chap. 8 of [1; includes citations].

We will consider this in more detail in Chapter 9 but, briefly, practically any male animal which feels challenged will show a preparatory surge of *testosterone*. If he wins the challenge, his testosterone levels will stay high or may even increase. The winner will strut around assertively, attracting attention and generally behaving in a dominant manner that is likely to provoke further challenges from nearby males. In the loser, however, levels of the hormone drop sharply and he will look and feel defeated. In non-human species, males will not normally react unless a challenge is directly perceived, mostly seeing, hearing or smelling another male. In humans, however, merely anticipating a challenge will produce the same effect. This has been shown many times in sportsmen. Starting some hours before the match, their levels of testosterone rise, peaking soon after the match starts. It declines after the match, slowly in the victor and rapidly in the loser, but the blood level goes up and down depending entirely on the outcome. If a man who thought he had lost wins on appeal, his testosterone levels will start to rise again. All of this is under direct mental control. There is no way it can be explained in non-mentalist terms.

We can explain it as a two-stage process. The first is the computational process of determining whether there is or isn't a challenge. A challenge is broadly defined as any event that could result in loss of status (including property, up to and including loss of life) because it is *loss of perceived status* that causes the fall in testosterone levels. From the computational point of view, this is relatively easy but we almost certainly have an innate capacity to guage threats, just as monkeys, dogs and birds do.

Once this decision is made, and remember it is very fast and not open to introspection, then signals are sent to a variety of brain centres which in turn activate a cascade of systems throughout the body. One of them is the fight or flight response, which we will look at in more detail in Sect. 6.7, and another is the testosterone circuits. The decision "I am being challenged," is computed by the ineffably complex prefrontal neuronal circuits. This decision is then directed to the specialised secretory neurons in the preoptic and suprachiasmatic regions of the hypothalamus. Neurologically, these are end-point neurons in that, while they receive spike impulses, they do not transmit them as they don't connect onwards to more neurons. Instead, their output takes the form of chemicals known as hormone releasing factors, chemicals which the body can "understand" (this means only that there is a specific receptor activated by just those chemicals). By this process, a thought ("I've really got to win this") is conveyed from the brain to a point where it is converted into physiological activity, thus bridging the physiological mind-body gap. In this respect, there is precious little difference between humans and most other animals. We will come back to this point in the final sections of this volume.

The neurosecretory neurons themselves represent no conceptual problems. In humans, *GNRH1*, the gene for gonadotrophin releasing factor (GnRH), is located on chromosome 8. It is activated to its expressive state by a specific pattern of neuronal impulses impinging on the cell body via a G-protein receptor chain. Once activated, *GNRH1* immediately causes production of the decapeptide releasing factor, which travels via the secretory neuron to the pituitary portal system and thence to the anterior pituitary. There, stored LH and FSH are released into the bloodstream to travel to their target, the testicular Leydig cells. By a similar process, testosterone is rapidly produced and secreted into the bloodstream, so that it can act upon its own target organs, including the brain. The critical structure here is probably the amygdala, which has long been implicated in aggressive behavior. All of this takes less than a minute. Subsequently, a further decision "Hooray, I've won" or "Oh no, I've lost," will either enhance or suppress the testosterone response, influencing the subject's behaviour accordingly.

This principle applies very widely throughout the human body. Western medicine has very little understanding of the feedback loops involved in homeostasis, but mostly because it rejects the notion that there is a causally-effective mind quietly pulling physiological strings. It is difficult to reconcile this blind spot with the everyday knowledge of the placebo effect but, as Lord Lister realised, people see only the facts supporting their point of view.

6.7 Output states: the path of emotional functions

Emotion is essentially psychiatry's home territory; all the more surprising, then, to learn that orthodox psychiatry doesn't have a model of emotion nor, indeed, any suggestions as to how it relates to cognition and physiology. As mentioned previously, the process of experiencing an emotion is not dissimilar to the process of experiencing ordinary sensations, except they are generated and perceived wholly internally. What we call emotions are simply internal sensations, albeit of a particular kind, but not different in principle from pain or hearing.

An experience of any kind requires an input, a receptor/transducer which converts the input into the currency of neurons, i.e. neuronal spike impulses, and a central data processor or interpreter, which manipulates the data flow to produce the particular experience. In the case of vision, the input is light energy; the transducers are the retinal photoreceptors which, alone in the body, convert light energy into nerve impulses, and the brain does the rest. In the biocognitive model, the input to whatever centres function to generate the emotional experience just is a cerebral outflow, meaning activating instructions from the higher executive centres to the emotional "equipment." In turn, its output is fed back to the cerebral cortex where, by the same principle outlined for exteroception, an experience of emotion is generated. This amounts to a recursive loop such that, even though we may not realise it at the time, we are ultimately responsible for our emotions. It is not a case of "choosing" to feel something (as in "That man frightens me." "Oh, you're just choosing to feel scared, you could be calm if you wanted to."), as our our emotions are determined by high-speed decisions relying on barely apprehended rules that often go back to early childhood.

Two emotions in particular will demonstrate these points, anxiety and depression.

6.8 Output states: anxiety

Anxiety is far and away the most powerful of all human emotions. It is the only truly recursive emotion, which explains its power, and is central to a great deal of behaviour in the sense of "life as a struggle to avoid anxiety." The concept of anxiety is quite simple: it is the body's internal alarm system, designed to save our bacon. Actually, it exists to save our genes but we have only recently realised we have such things so, for millions of years, anxiety has quietly done its job without anybody knowing what it was for. The perception of a threat activates the alarm system which prepares the individual to deal with the threat ("fight or flight").

The cognitive act of perceiving a threat is necessary and sufficient to produce an anxiety response. That is, anxiety is always and only the response to the perception of a threat. Nothing else can do it. A threat is always in the future, coming toward us. We cannot be frightened of the past. We may be angry about it, amused by it, grief-stricken or bored by the past but we can't be scared of it. We can only be scared of what is coming our way, of the looming danger that has to be avoided if we want to see tomorrow.

All animals experience anxiety or something very similar, unless they are armour-plated, like abalone, and even they have a defensive reaction when touched. The neural mechanism that subserves the experience of emotion is wired into the brain, closely associated with the hippocampus and amygdala, and is practically the same in all animals studied. This indicates that, in evolutionary terms, anxiety is very old, which further indicates how successful it has been in doing its job of saving the very genes that program for it.

The decision "There is a threat" is computed by the highest centres as a simple cognitive assessment. There is a strong innate element as well, in that certain perceptions are more likely to provoke anxiety than others (any elementary textbook of psychology will describe these). Once the decision is made, it is instantly relayed to thalamic, brainstem and other structures which implement the instruction, alerting the entire body to be ready to deal with the threat. This is the "flight or fight" reaction which has a number of components. The first is the familiar physical constellation of somatic symptoms including shaking, sweating, churning stomach, racing heart, shortness of breath, dry mouth, tightness in the throat, light-headedness and stammering speech.

Associated with these symptoms are various cognitive changes, in that the mind seems to spin faster and faster, dragging in possibilities that ordinarily wouldn't be considered, until there are too many thoughts tumbling through the head. Some people experience the opposite, complaining that their mind goes blank and they can't think what they have to do. In addition, there are perceptual changes such as a feeling of being trapped, commonly described as "the walls closing in," and the sense that the world somehow looks different, or the person himself feels different, either from others or from his normal self. These are the classic anxiety symptoms of depersonalisation and derealisation. They are most emphatically *not* symptoms of something else called "dissociation."

These features of the anxiety response, both somatic and cognitive, don't require much explanation, except on one point: very often, they reinforce themselves. That is, there can be a positive feedback loop which intensifies the somatic symptoms to the point of complete panic. People can become scared of their own anxiety symptoms, as in: There is nothing to fear but fear itself.

The first group, the familiar physical changes, get the body ready to deal with the threat, either by fighting or by running away. The second group, the cognitive changes, are mediated by the ascending reticular activating system in the brain stem. This projects to the whole cortex and shifts brain function several notches higher, as it were. It is activated either by instructions from above, or by peripheral sensory input itself, such as being touched unexpectedly. In the state of heightened arousal, the person is thinking rapidly of ways to deal with the threat, face it or avoid it. As long as he perceives he is at risk, his mind will throw up more and more outlandish suggestions. Commonly, these relate to the cause of the threat, as in who is behind it, and these paranoid ideas can themselves be frightening, which reinforces his fear state, leading to panic. During high anxiety, the separate cognitive functions of concentration (attention) and memory are affected, leading to concentration and memory defects.

Finally, there is the subjective sense of fear, the sense of dread or impending doom that, for a sufferer, is the core of the emotion. The model says that the cognitive decision "There is a threat" activates certain subcortical centres, which then feed their activity back to the cortical regions, thereby generating a perception via the same or a very similar mechanism as that proposed for exteroception in Sect. 6.4. Note that the expression "There is a threat" is only a description of what happens, not a formal explanation. Language as we understand it is not involved, the decision is made at a subverbal level. People jump before they know why they are jumping, and certainly before they could possibly put the concept into mental "words." The anxiety reaction is very fast. It has to be, because nature doesn't give second chances.

It isn't possible to experience an anxiety reaction without the perception of a threat. Nobody can say: "I'm bored, I think I'll have a nice panic attack to liven the day." The generic concept of threat, whatever that is, is immutably tied to the anxiety response. We may try to overrule it, to control the anxiety by willpower, but it doesn't work: if you have perceived a threat, your heart will start to race. If your heart isn't racing, it means you have somehow managed to neutralise the perception so that it no longer appears threatening. Anxiety always has a cause, it has an "about." It is whatever idea provoked the agitation but it is often so fast and so fleeting that the frightened person, whose memory may not be working very well at the time, doesn't recall it. There is no such thing as "free-floating anxiety," a cliche which means only that the psychiatrist hasn't taken a proper history.

The problem for humans is that the symptoms of anxiety can become a threat in their own right. This opens the way to the concept of a recursive loop of anxiety, a self-reinforcing state which can only intensify. For example, for whatever reason, the heart may accelerate a little. The person then becomes anxious about just this, as in "Oh no, I'm about to have a heart attack," or, more commonly, "Oh no, this is going to turn into a really bad panic, I just know it. Help help." This is why humans can have panic attacks but animals can't.

Anxiety is real and immensely powerful. It has to be because, in the final analysis, it is the emotion that guarantees our survival. Anxiety is not, in any valid or plausible sense of the term, an illness or disease. It is the human body doing exactly what it has been programmed to do by millions of years of evolution. The concept of anxiety as a recursive informational state is developed in [5].

6.9 Output states: depression

Depression is now deemed one of the most costly burdens of illness in the world. I propose that the principle outlined for anxiety also applies in the case of misery except, where the triggering decision in anxiety is "I see a threat," in depression, the triggering decision is "I have suffered a loss." In order to explain this, we have to assume that the concept of loss is generic, i.e. it applies to losses such as losing another person, goods, territory, health, status... anything. That is, before we can experience the sense of loss, we must have formed an emotional bond to the object, whatever it is. When the bond is abruptly broken, the reaction is the sense of misery and despair we call grief. If and when a grief reaction occurs without an obvious loss, we say the person is depressed but the emotional states and all other changes involved are exactly the same. As phenomena, grief and depression differ in name only.

Different authors approach grief in different ways but most people now accept the broad outline of grief as a more or less stereotyped process, attributed to the Swiss physician, Elisabeth Kübler-Ross (1926–2004). She saw the grieving person proceeding through five stages, beginning with a short-lived phase of shock and denial [6]. This is followed by a phase in which anger is the dominant emotion, then bargaining, followed by depression and acceptance. These stages are not, of course, pure or delineated by recognisable cut-off points. They blur as people move back and forth while slowly progressing toward the goal, which is recovery and a new lifestyle separate from the loss.

As we normally use the term, depression is somewhat different in that it develops slowly, over months, weeks or even days, but with no obvious cause. Of course, if there were an obvious cause, we wouldn't call it depression. Otherwise, the phenomena of grief and depression are the same. The central feature of the two syndromes is the loss of any form of joy or positive emotion. People can no longer experience happiness from everything they once found pleasurable or rewarding. Events they once liked just because they were pleasurable seem empty, devoid of interest or joy, and pointless. As the mood intensifies, everything comes to seem useless and hopeless, and their feelings towards themselves veer toward a sense of helplessness and despair. They start to feel that if this is life, there is no point, it will never get better so it may as well end now. In a small proportion of cases, that is just what happens.

If, however, they can wait long enough, which the great majority of people do, slowly, without any other changes, their mood starts to lift. Colours start to seem bright again, while happy sounds such as music, birds calling or children laughing stop grating. The taste of food returns, minor irritations seem bearable, sex starts to seem more than just an empty biological exercise, and the future seems a little less bleak. The whole process of a grief reaction or a depressive state lasts from four to eight months or longer, and seriously interrupts life, occasionally leading to its end.

We humans survive just because we can form bonds. Perhaps the downside of bonds is the grief we experience when they are broken, but we would not be the same creatures without them. Grief and depression are one and the same emotion. Depression is not, in any valid sense of the term, an illness or disease. It is the human body doing exactly what it has been programmed to do by millions of years of evolution. It can be understood in terms of the computational or bio-cognitive model of mind, using the same concepts as for anxiety.

It is a given in this model that emotions are mediated by specific but complex brain structures, even though we have only the most superficial knowledge of what they are and how they work. It is clear that the experience of pleasure involves particular pathways, many of which focus on the nucleus accumbens in the anterior forebrain. However, it must not be thought that there is a "pleasure centre." It is probably reasonable to say there are "pleasure circuits" in the brain, activation of which is necessary and sufficient for the experience of pleasure. That is, a decision is made in the executive centres along the lines "That was very good." Immediately, instructions are relayed to these "pleasure circuits," activating them. In turn, they send a flow of data back to the cortex where it is received and, by some recursive algorithmic processing, the experience of happiness is generated. At this stage, that is all we can say; it is also all we need to say.

The experience "I have suffered a loss" is computed by the highest centres as a simple cognitive assessment, although there is also a strong innate element (insofar as the concept of affective bonds is innate). Computationally, this is a very simple matter, as in:

> Once, I had that object.
> It was important to me.
> Now, I don't have it.
> Therefore, I have suffered a loss.

Once the decision of loss is made, instructions are relayed to the deeper brainstem and other structures which subserve the experience of pleasure, causing an inhibitory block of just these circuits. That is, an awareness of loss paralyses the pleasure centres so that further instructions are ineffective. This is a normal, natural process, genetically-determined and fully comprehensible by standard scientific methods. It is not a disease process. The unhappy subject now has to get through life deprived of any joy, amusement, wonder, everything that makes daily life feel worthwhile. Instead of being lifted up a dozen times a day, he sinks slowly into a state of *unjoy*, cut off from his peers who can't understand why he is unable to share their happiness.

It is possible that the cortical signal which inhibits the basal brain centres is a single event which produces long-lasting changes in synaptic transmission but it seems more likely that, after a loss, these centres are bombarded by dozens, even hundreds of signals a day, with a new one generated each time the unhappy individual is reminded of the loss. If each signal produces 15 minutes of inhibition, which is physiologically more likely, it doesn't take many signals per day to lead to total loss of pleasure. Gradually, as the grieving person develops a new life, the awareness of loss diminishes, the blockade fades and life slowly returns to normal.

In the case of a grief reaction, we don't know how to accelerate recovery but we certainly do know how to make it worse. If, after suffering a bereavement, the individual can't establish a satisfying lifestyle, then the grieving process will seem to go on and on. Since grief is not an illness (so far, although psychiatrists are trying to turn it into one), no treatment is required. Friends and relatives simply need to provide a sheltered and supportive environment while the bereaved person journeys through the preordained process of the grief reaction until, in the fullness of time, he emerges at the other side, ready to resume life. If he can't progress, then something is blocking his recovery, and needs to be explored. Sometimes, it is obvious, like a desperately unhappy marriage, or it may be more subtle, like an unsuspected anxiety state. Constant anxiety destroys any sense that life can ever be any good; a person who comes to this realisation will soon sink into despair and anhedonia, otherwise known as "depression." But if the anxiety component isn't recognised and managed, he will never feel he has a future and cannot recover. The only reason anxiety isn't recognised is because nobody asked the right questions.

6.10 Conclusion

All too often, we hear people say things like "Mind and brain are a unity," or "Mind and brain are identical." Such comments are just a weak attempt to side-step the crucial questions in philosophy of mind, and they fail. If mind and brain are identical, they must have all their properties in common, which is manifestly untrue: I can see something blue as a mental event, or even a memory of blue, but be assured there is nothing blue in my brain. The brain is the mechanism for the implementation of the mind, but mind can never be reduced to its mechanism.

David Chalmers splits the problem of consciousness in two, the easy and hard problems of consciousness. The easy problem is the notion of decision-making or executive functions. The solution proposed here goes back to the startingly original work of the mathematician, George Boole, and develops through some of the most brilliant minds of the twentieth century. Decisions are made using a Boolean-type algebra, implemented on logic gates coded into the walls of neurons. Apart from the bit about logic gates, that is all fairly unremarkable. These days, we do not have a problem with non-mentalist decision-making. Johnson-Laird's dictum that any scientific theory of the mind must treat it as an automaton is no longer frightening.

A definitive solution to the hard problem of consciousness remains elusive but I don't believe that means we must give up. Instead, the solution proposed here is that mental life is implemented by the same neural architecture as is used to make decisions, albeit with different forms of processing. This will be true for all animals that have similar neural structures, meaning essentially all creatures on earth, but most emphatically for the more complex mammals, including marine mammals. Because the neural structures are so widely distributed in nature, we assume that they arose very early in evolution, certainly by the end of the Cambrian Explosion starting 540 million years ago. That actually tells us a lot and, I believe, has profound moral implications for how humans treat animals (without starting on the question of how humans treat other humans).

Putting those matters aside, the proposed solution to the hard problem of consciousness, meaning explaining the actual experience of mental life, relies on recursive processing of both sensory (exogenous) and emotional (endogenous) data. The algorithms or processing instructions by which this is achieved are completely unknown, except we can be fairly sure they are largely generated by experience, just because there isn't enough information in the human genome to code for that level of complexity. That is, early life experience becomes critically important in understanding how and why the mind develops but it also indicates the processing routines are likely to be clever and subtle rather than prodigiously complex. This may not be cause for optimism but at least it suggests where we should look. Or maybe it just tells us where we should stop looking, as in looking for "chemical imbalances in the brain."

References

[1] McLaren N (2007) Behaviorism from the psychiatric perspective. Chapter 3 in McLaren N (2007) *Humanizing Madness: Psychiatry and the Cognitive Neurosciences.*; Ann Arbor, Mi.: Future Psychiatry Press.

[2] Forsyth M (2013) *The Elements of Eloquence: how to turn the perfect English phrase.* London: Icon Books.

[3] McLaren N (2012). Testing the biocognitive model: Testosterone and the Challenge Hypothesis. Chapter 8 in *The Mind-Body Problem Explained: The Biocognitive Model for Psychiatry.* Ann Arbor, MI: Future Psychiatry Press.

[4] Stoljar D (2010). *Physicalism.* Oxford: Routledge.

[5] McLaren N (2018). *Anxiety: The Inside Story.* Ann Arbor, MI: Future Psychiatry Press.

[6] Kübler-Ross E (1969). *On Death & Dying,* New York: Simon & Schuster/ Touchstone.

7 Implementing dualism: fundamental principles

The brain is a product of evolution, and just as animal brains have their limitations, we have ours. Our brains can't hold a hundred numbers in memory, can't visualize seven-dimensional space and perhaps can't intuitively grasp why neural information processing, observed from the outside, should give rise to subjective experience on the inside.

Stephen Pinker (b. 1954)

We know that people can maintain an unshakable faith in any proposition, however absurd, when they are sustained by a community of like-minded believers

Daniel Kahneman (b. 1934)
Thinking, Fast and Slow (2011)

As our own species is in the process of proving, one cannot have superior science and inferior morals. The combination is unstable and self-destroying.
Arthur C Clarke (1917–2008)

7.1 The formal basis of dualism

The goal in this chapter is to draw the case together by deriving a formal basis for a dualist model of mind. We start with the definition of information in Sect.4.2:

7.1.1 *Information* is an assessment of some discernible aspect of the universe by an entity with the capacity to represent states of affairs in a symbolic calculus.

As mentioned previously, there is a strong circular element in this definition, which relates to the self-evident fact that only an entity with a prodigious informational capacity can comprehend that definition. As we proceed with this chapter, this particular problem will recur. Unfortunately, we are so accustomed to seeing the universe from our vantage point as information processors that we tend to forget how remarkable it is. We think, for example, that colours inhere in objects but they don't. There are no colours, no sounds, no tastes or smells in the material universe unless and until the relevant energy pattern is discerned and

DOI: 10.4324/9781003183792-7

processed by "....an entity with the capacity to represent states of affairs in a symbolic calculus."

> *Sensations and knowledge inhere in the mental state of a minded being, not in the object itself.*

An apple isn't red until you see it, the sky isn't blue until you look up, but because it's always blue when we look up, we start to think it's blue even when we can't see it. Because microwave radiation is colourless, those beautiful pictures of distant galaxies are the product of colours photoshopped on to digital arrays collected by radio-telescopes. Since our entire lives are based on our perceptions of the external world, and since these are so reliable and predictable, we assume that what we see is what is there. This is an example of the *projectionist fallacy*, the error of projecting our perceptions to the world and then assuming they are inherent and objectively independent of us.

7.1.2 *Computation* is the manipulation of information according to the rules of a symbolic calculus coded in a physical system with sufficient switching capacity.

Information is worthless until we do something with it. Prior to the discovery of the Rosetta Stone, for Europeans, Egyptian hieroglyphs were just decoration, pretty noise. Doing something with information, even reading it to commit to memory, is a form of computation.

7.1.3 A *physical system* implements a given computation when the causal structure of the physical system mirrors the formal structure of the computation (Chalmers).

This has been covered in more detail in **S.2.3-2.5**. It builds on the work of Turing and of Shannon, who saw the parallels between the input-output states of truth tables for some of the basic logic functions, and certain precisely configured switching devices. What Definition **7.1.3** says is just what Shannon determined from basic principles in his Masters thesis, that there is a precise relationship between the calculus of propositions and symbolic relay analysis. If a set of switches is built to mirror the specifications of a dual-valued logic, it functions as a little logic device, or logic gate. Given these enormous intellectual leaps by far-sighted individuals, the path to a dualist model of mind becomes clear.

Critically, the consumption of energy by a logic gate does not determine its output. A gate uses no more energy to compute its response than if it opens and closes randomly, computing nothing. Once a system of switches is operating, once energy is being expended shunting data around the circuits, computation is a free lunch.

7.1.4 An *informational state* is the total informational content of an implemented computation at a particular instant.

This point is important for a theory of mental disorder. The outcome of any computational process depends on the total informational input. It may be possible after the event to state that some part of the process was not necessary in arriving at the decision (as in 3+2-2=3) but that assumes the observer has full knowledge of all the steps involved, which is only true in idealised systems. In poorly-defined systems, such as biological or other naturally-occurring mechanisms, the observer can only have a rough indication of the major factors involved. Any attempt to restrict the significance of an informational state is arbitrary. Significantly for psychiatry, any attempt to separate an informational state from its previous states, or its consequences, is arbitrary.

Corollary 7.1.4.1: Informational states can be instantaneous or extended over time.

An informational state extended over time is an *informational space.*

7.1.5 A *mental state* is an informational state implemented in a physical system with sufficient switching capacity to acquire and instantiate particular recursive properties leading to the emergence of perceptual awareness.

Corollary 7.1.5.1: Not all physical switching systems implement mental states, i.e. conscious awareness is not universal (as in panpsychism).

This defines a mental state and restricts its occurrence in nature to certain highly-developed systems. Trees do not have the switching capacity to allow mental states to develop. The nematode *Caenorhabditis elegans* has 302 neurons and about 7000 neuronal connections, which seems far too small to undertake the sorts of computations needed for the emergence of mental properties such as conscious awareness. The sea-slug *Aplysia californica* has 10-20,000 neurons but still seems to operate at the very crudest S-R level. Nonetheless, we can't say that it doesn't selectively choose what it eats or react aversively to noxious (painful) stimuli, so we can't say it doesn't have basic sensory experiences. When we compare the neural machinery and behaviour of fish, reptiles, birds and mammals, increasingly, the similarities outweigh the differences. At this stage of our knowledge, it is impossible, if not absurd, to claim that only humans enjoy conscious awareness.

Corollary 7.1.5.2: Mental states cannot exist independently of a suitable physical switching system, i.e. there is *no disembodied conscious awareness.*

Corollary 7.1.5.2 excludes anything we would traditionally regard as supernatural.

7.1.6 A mental state is an element of the set of all informational states.

Corollary 7.1.6.1: A mental state exists by virtue of its being a representation of a state of affairs, i.e. by being an informational state.

Corollary 7.1.6.2: There is no mentality without information, or content-free mental states.

This reiterates that a dualist mentality is both real and wholly a natural matter, but also points to the directedness of information. That is, information is always and only *about* something (a state of affairs), which settles the question of intensionality of mental states. If a mental state isn't about something, then it isn't a mental state. Corollary 7.1.6.1 confirms that there can't be a mental state about nothing. If we are awake, we are aware of something. Corollary 7.1.6.2 excludes that favorite of mystics, the oxymoron of pure consciousness, or consciousness devoid of content.

7.1.7   Necessarily, the causative context of a mental state is part of the implemented computation that constitutes the emergent informational space, so a particular mental state cannot be considered separately from its context.

Any attempt to present a particular mental element as "free-standing," "free-floating3 or independent of the totality of the informational state of the individual is neither empirical nor *a priori*. It is arbitrary, and therefore non-scientific. Biological psychiatry defines mental symptoms as *sui generis*, mental in name only and independent of context or meaning. In their view, the informational content of a mental symptom is restricted to its status as an indicator of pathology at the level of the genome. A depressed mood, for example, is held to be biological brute fact. It does not require explanation in terms of "meaning" in the subject's life as the informational content of a depressed mood relates to the genome only. In turn, genetic "facts" are held to be completely independent of life experiences, which exemplifies the perfectly circular justification of biological psychiatry.

In a fully-developed reductionist biological psychiatry, mental symptoms are divorced from the context of the individual's life, and only a specialist can understand their significance. Since the ordinary human knows nothing about genomes, his life history and his mental symptoms are held to exist as separate informational sets. To the biological psychiatrist, the individual's life history has no conceivable bearing on his symptoms because they are biological facts which were set in motion at the moment of conception. Of course, this claim is immediately refuted by daily experience.

7.1.8   A mental state of one individual can be conveyed to another, suitably equipped individual by means of an agreed code, or language.

Language allows the listener to recreate in his own mind a facsimile of the informational content of the speaker's mind. If speaker and audience have an agreed code and a physical medium for transfer of the physical patterns used to convey the information (air, paper, wifi), then Shannon's conditions of communication (see

Sect.2.5) are satisfied: "The fundamental problem of communication is that of reproducing at one point either exactly or approximately a message selected at another point." In order to convert mere communication into language, he qualified this: "Frequently the messages have meaning; that is they refer to or are correlated according to some system with certain physical or conceptual entities." That is, if speaker and audience have agreed on what the messages signify, then the audience "knows what the speaker means." If there isn't agreement, things go awry. For example, the Thai word ฟัก sounds exactly like a certain vulgar English word. At a roadside stall once, the pretty young girl selling vegetables smiled sweetly and asked me คุณต้องการฟักไหม? Startled, I turned to the student with me, who laughed and explained: "She ask if you want *pumpkin*." The impression created in my mind by that phoneme was *not* a facsimile of what she had in her mind. Shannon understood this: "These semantic aspects of communication are irrelevant to the engineering problem." They are certainly not irrelevant to human relations.

Armed with these basic points, we can consider some of the more salient "design constraints" of a dualist model of mind.

7.2 Physiological Constraints

Previous chapters have outlined the case for the mind being a causally-effective informational "space" generated by the very proficient, biological data processor called the brain. This is a hypothetical construct: while we can say an informational space is not part of the material universe, we cannot yet specify it in more detail. There are, however, certain basic principles that must be taken into account before the concept of a brain-based informational state makes any sense.

The first principle is that the brain is an extremely delicate organ that operates between exceedingly narrow physiological limits. Some people find this a bit shocking; after all, doesn't my brain kick into gear every morning when I wake up? Indeed, but there's a lot of unseen work that goes into that quotidian wonder. If the chemical bath in which the brain floats varies even slightly from its normal state, then it begins to malfunction. Any slight variation in the plasma electrolytes, blood gases or glucose level, or many other metabolites, can produce a disturbance of brain function manifest as impairments of conscious level or conscious content. Drugs, of course, can seriously interfere with the brain, the most common of all being alcohol, but there are many others. Concussion, high fevers and systemic infections typically impair mental function while metabolic illnesses such as diabetes, uraemia or hepatic failure are equally well-known to affect conscious function. A whole range of metals, organic chemicals and the like are known to produce the clinical picture of confusion (cognitive impairment). There is, however, no evidence that these or any other chemicals or physical disturbances can reliably reproduce (as distinct from contributing to or complicating) the standard psychiatric syndromes. We will come back to this point later.

7.3 Modularity

Reprising Sect.3.4, the brain is composed of a large number of functionally distinct modules whose informational output combines to produce the effect of being a thinking, feeling, experiencing individual with a personal history. The great Russian neuropsychologist Aleksandr Luria (1902-77) wrote insightfully on this; his work remains a classic today [1]. Each *module* must be explained in full. It is important to be acutely aware that the total conscious state (of being oneself) is not a true unity but is an artefact generated by the interaction of dozens, even hundreds, of functionally distinct mental entities. We tend to take the unity of conscious experience for granted because it always seems to work so effortlessly but again, there's a lot of work going on behind the scenes to keep that impression on track. In certain conditions, even as slight as lack of sleep, their apparently seamless function can start to disintegrate, which can be terrifying to the patient and his relatives and, all too often, confusing to the psychiatrist.

7.4 Arousal

The concept of *arousal* is critically important. Arousal is a physiological measure of the brain's total state of alertness. Arousal measures the parameter that ranges from sleep to drowsiness to alertness to over-alertness. There is a very clear relationship, known as the *Yerkes-Dodson curve*, between performance (on any task) and arousal. At low levels of arousal, as when we are waking in the morning, performance is poor but, as the arousal level lifts, performance improves. It then reaches a plateau, after which any further increase in arousal results in loss of performance, shown at Pt 7 on the graph below (Figure 7.1). This is the stage of "mental breakdown," although it really should be called performance breakdown: (Figure 7.1)

In general, we tend to equate arousal and anxiety but it's not entirely accurate. A person can be highly aroused with no anxiety at all (playing sport, winning something or achieving a major goal), or can be on the verge of sleep while still decidedly anxious, but it's a good enough approximation. In practice, the most common cause of high arousal is anxiety (the response to a threat) but depressed people are also highly aroused. Early morning waking is a sign of over-arousal, most commonly due to anxiety but also seen in severe depressive states. It is not a sign of depression per se. Panic states, of course, are examples of excessively high arousal and an acutely psychotic person is also highly aroused even if he appears to be obtunded or even stuporose. The highest arousal of all is seen in catatonia, either the stupor or excitement. Acute stuporose catatonia is treated by infusing an anesthetising dose of a tranquilliser, or even an anesthetic agent, such as sodium pentothal. The patient "wakes up," a trick which always startles medical students. Fortunately, this condition is now unusual in western populations although it will still be seen in recent immigrants, especially from developing countries:

The critical point is that the brain's modular functions integrate smoothly only within a narrow band of arousal (shown on the graph between x=5-8). That is,

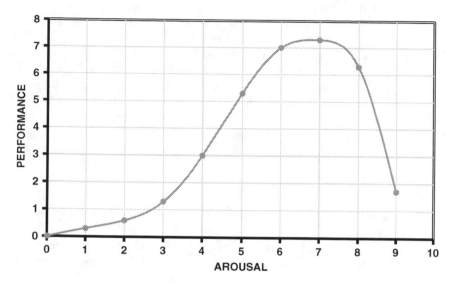

Figure 7.1 Yerkes-Dodson Curve.

the mind exists as a seamless entity only while the brain is operating within narrow physiological limits. Below normal arousal, as when we are waking up in the morning or over-tired, or above it for any reason, the separate modular functions start to split apart. Memory, for example, doesn't work well at either extreme; if somebody gives you a message when you are overtired, you are likely to forget it in a few minutes. At the other extreme, you can give perfectly clear instructions to a very frightened person and he will have them jumbled up almost before you have finished speaking. This may also be partly because attention and concentration begin to malfunction after relatively slight changes in arousal. Motor functions lose their smooth integration at both ends of the scale: tired people bump into things and agitated people drop things.

At the highest levels of arousal, core functions such as the senses of familiarity and novelty begin to malfunction. They may switch on or off unpredictably, so a familiar object may seem strange or different, or something novel may seem very familiar. These effects can happen briefly in normal life (deja vu, jamais vu) and we don't worry about them but, to an over-aroused person, the effects can be sustained and become terrifying in themselves. Not uncommonly, highly aroused people start to hallucinate. What are sometimes called stress-induced hallucinations do not equate to a formal psychotic condition, although they must be taken seriously. The essential feature is that high arousal produces mental effects which serve to frighten patients more, making them even more highly aroused, which produces further disturbance in a self-perpetuating cycle, or vicious circle.

It is vital for psychiatrists to be familiar with all manifestations of high arousal; recognising it and dealing with it effectively is an essential part of daily practice.

One of the best places to see cases of high arousal is in the emergency department. It isn't just the patients or their relatives who are excessively aroused, but also medical or nursing staff, police and other support staff. We will come back to this point but one of the most basic and important skills to learn is how to recognise over-arousal and to talk the patient down to some level of normality. Talking to a frightened adult is no different from talking to a frightened child or frightened animal. The same rule applies in each case: don't shout or act in a threatening manner or you will make them worse. If you act in a threatening manner, of if the person perceives you are acting in a threatening manner, he will become more aroused and may respond according to the threat he perceives.

7.5 Recursion

Recursion is the capacity for something to act back upon itself. A recursive mathematical formula is one which takes the outcome of its first iteration as the starting point for its second iteration. In medicine, we tend to think of recursion as the various types of biochemical and physiological processes that act to maintain the *milieu interieur*, or physiological *homeostasis*. At the biochemical level, thousands of these processes have been described in a myriad species. Everything about the body is designed to keep it functioning within specified limits, because anything outside those limits either consumes too much energy or is potentially dangerous. This also applies to the mental state.

Normally, we try to keep ourselves pleasantly comfortable with occasional bursts of controlled excitement such as football games, bungie jumping or a bit of light-hearted speeding, but a little bit of arousal goes a long way. If arousal moves too far from normality, the mental state starts to deteriorate rapidly. There are many, many mental mechanisms whose role is to maintain an equable state. However, these mechanisms break down in recognisable ways under specific stressors.

Very often, mental disorders are *self-reinforcing*, the clearest example being anxiety. If a person becomes aroused to the point where his heart starts to race, he may then start to think he is about to have a heart attack. This idea itself intensifies his anxiety, which makes his heart beat faster still, and may lead to a full panic state. The concept of mental disorders as states of self-reinforcing abnormality is central to the biocognitive model for psychiatry. Pathology acts recursively: an abnormal mental state acts back upon itself to intensify the abnormality. This can be confusing for the observer (not to mention the unfortunate patient) but recognising it is critical for daily practice as standard (drug) treatment will often make it worse. The goal of treatment is to negate the self-reinforcing element in the developing abnormal state, in order to break the vicious circle.

This feature is central to the concept that the presence of mental disorder says nothing about the biological state of the brain. Mental disorder is the result of the brain doing precisely what it is meant to do, except it can get out of control, not as a matter of biology but as a predictable matter of information processing.

7.6 Evolutionary influences

Evolution shapes our destinies. This is complicated and we will revisit the principle at different points, but our evolutionary history is far more powerful than we would like to admit. In general, our prodigious intellectual ability is the servant of our worst drives, not the master (see Clarke's quote above; also [2]). Granted, this leads to a pessimistic view of humans but anybody who doubts it need only look at the evening news to realise its truth. There is a basis for this within the biocognitive model, but it also suggests a solution.

7.7 Conflicting drives

This is a loose cluster of features that also stem from our evolutionary heritage, but they are not always compatible. Therefore, it is a toss-up as to which one wins at any time. Within the mind, our intellectual or knowledge-based functions take a welter of information from a wide range of external and internal sources and integrate it almost instantaneously to give a single course of action. All of this is done at a level we can't access but it is still our personal decision. If it were any different, we wouldn't survive. In the main, we make rapid but cautious and conservative decisions. Many of our fears seem to have a strong innate basis. Frogs, for example, are among the most harmless creatures on earth, yet huge numbers of people are terrified of them, a fear which starts very early in life, long before any training could have taken place. Cognitively, we have many innate biases that need to be explored in detail [e.g. 3].

Like most animals, we are creatures of habit, but we have our own evolutionary imperatives. First and foremost, we are social animals. Clustering in groups has a variety of outcomes but the driving force is that it feels better than being isolated. Isolation is frightening to the point of being mentally destabilising (see Yerkes-Dodson curve above). Once established, groups are held together by affectionate bonds, a powerful emotional reinforcer that generally over-rides rationality. Familiar faces are reassuring while strangers are unsettling, a cause for apprehension and uncertainty. *Xenophobia* is the opposite side of the coin to our version of the social drive. The combination of social and xenophobic drives leads to *tribalism*, which is one of our worst characteristics.

No sooner do humans form their little social groups than they establish *dominance* hierarchies, both within their groups and between them. Practically all primates do this. Some people like to be leaders, but most are happy to be led, as it provokes less anxiety. For the majority, the thought of doing something wrong inhibits any urge to be the alpha male or female. For a few in every group, holding power wins every time: somebody else can always be blamed when things go wrong. There is a very powerful physiological reason behind the hierarchical urge, we'll come back to it.

Next, our little groups show *territoriality*: we are territorial. We like to acquire space and property and we guard them jealously. We are pre-programmed to acquire but, because this drive developed when resources were very limited, we don't actually know when to stop. Early in our evolution, we had no need for a Stop button, so we don't have one. Having more feels better than not having any (is this the basis of the notion of the harem?). All over the world, *inequality* is increasing daily, dragging with it a multitude of psychological, social and environmental ills, and all because we are innately biased against saying "Enough is enough." Again, territoriality fits with the notion of dominance hierarchies.

Like most apes, we are curious creatures, given to exploring and creating. We like to see what is in the next valley or around the bend of the river. We like to look inside, to climb on, take apart, to build and change, to collect and to decorate. We like to *play* but sometimes the play gets too serious and spills over into our most characteristic and most damaging feature, *aggression*. Alone of all animals, we are boundlessly aggressive. Sometimes we use aggression instrumentally, to achieve goals, but mostly we fight because it feels good. Aggression becomes an end in itself. We actually like fighting and we certainly don't have any idea when to stop. On this point, we never learn. Aggression is not an illness, it is due to the brain doing exactly what the mind tells it to do, but the mind is biased in ways we don't fully understand – and don't want to know about.

7.8 Rationality

The next point concerns that Great Illusion, human *rationality*. From the point of view of the biocognitive model, there are two sides to this question, the first being the issues subsumed by Chalmers' "easy question of consciousness." That is, do we have the capacity to act in a rational manner? Yes, we do, and here is an example: 2+2=4. We must then ask: Do we have the neural machinery to perform rational acts? The model proposes a specific mechanism (logic gates coded into the walls of neurons) that supports an algorithmic computational process that can generate solutions to such problems. This is the basis to what we see as our prodigious rationality.

There is a history to this, of course. By the latter part of the nineteenth century, groups of grumpy old white men were fairly sure that they had the world sorted. Humans were the pinnacle of creation and white Protestant men stood at the pinnacle of humanity, therefore of creation, just a notch below the Almighty Himself - as determined by white Protestant men, of course. Men's steely, incisive minds had shown that the universe is a rational place that we can understand by applying the principles of mechanics and Newtonian physics, with some squishy bits for biology. This led to the *modernist illusion*, that the world is a place of infinite potential which we can harness to satisfy our every whim.

To late Victorian men, everything made sense, and by carefully applying our infallible minds to understanding the laws of the smoothly humming machinery of the universe, we could use it to satisfy our needs and impulses for ever. This is the instrumentalist view, that we can manipulate the universe as an instrument to satisfy our wishes (or we can act upon the universe as instruments to achieve our goals, same outcome). We were, indeed, Masters of the Universe. God? Of course there's always room for God, He (male) started it and set it up in such a sensible manner for us to exercise dominion over the beasts of the land and the fowls and fishes, not to mention women, children and the coloured races, who weren't always that easy to tell apart. For God's foresight and industry, He deserved our thanks (for an hour at eleven on Sundays, weather and the grouse season permitting).

There is just enough truth in this to allow us to delude ourselves, which leads to the dark side of the question of rationality. Yes, we can build giant cities with vast freeways so people can drive their luxurious cars from far distant suburbs and get to work on time; we can organise huge and hugely expensive spectacles like the Olympic Games that run like clockwork; we are very clever at building thermonuclear weapons and hurling them through space to destroy our enemies on the far side of the planet. We are just not good at deciding whether we should do these sorts of things. The whole truth is that our prodigious intellectual ability, our rationality, is not under rational control, it is the servant of some very base drives, not their master. There is a clear explanation for this in the bio-cognitive model; we will return to this point in Chapter 9.

7.9 Mental disorder

The other aspect of the rationality of the mind is that *mental disorder* makes sense. A rational machine can only malfunction in certain ways. A proper understanding of the brain and its emergent mind allows us to understand how and why it malfunctions, and to predict what is likely to happen. It is true that, just like any very complex machine, the brain can malfunction. That does not mean that every malfunction of the mind is necessarily due to a brain malfunction. Most emphatically, I am *not* saying that a full understanding of the brain will tell us all we need to know about human behaviour. That is not just wrong, it is absurd.

On the one hand, we have the tangible, physical machine of the brain, the one anaesthetists, neurologists and pathologists deal with. That particular machine functions in a certain way and it makes no difference whether it is awake or asleep, it still consumes energy while it gets on with its job. Anything that expends energy to work against the laws of thermodynamics can go wrong. The only processes that can't go wrong are processes driven by those laws, such as a bushfire, an avalanche, the water cycle or putrefaction. Because it consumes energy to work against the laws of thermodynamics, the brain can malfunction. It does so in certain predictable ways. *Epilepsy* is a physiological malfunction of the brain which, in terms of the brain's structure and function, makes perfect neurological sense. But neurology is not psychiatry.

The mind is not part of the physical structure of the brain, nor is it reducible to that structure. It emerges from the brain's functional architecture but is then independent of the brain and, within limits, is causally effective over the brain. It is governed by non-material laws, but it is still a rule-abiding entity. Therefore, it can and does malfunction. I have mentioned the two major sources of non-material errors that lead to mental disorder, errors in the input data set or errors in the computational algorithms. Either can produce an error in output, or what we call mental disorder.

A reductionist who claims that all mental disorder is necessarily brain disorder has set himself two very difficult tasks. The first is to show just how the physical brain produces mental disorder, while the second is the even more difficult task of proving that primary mental disorder is impossible. That is, in order to justify the reductionist claim, he has to prove that mental disorder cannot be the result of prior mental causes. When it is put this way, it is an impossible task, as the example of post-traumatic mental disorders shows. Insofar as the brain has an informational processing capacity, primary errors of that capacity are not just logically possible but, in real life, are highly likely.

Is this claim just another case of unfettered conceit, of "…carefully applying our infallible minds to understanding the laws of the smoothly humming machinery…" of the mind? I don't believe so, but the proof of this particular pudding lies in whether it works. Orthodox psychiatry doesn't work. Sorry, I'll rephrase that. Orthodox psychiatry works very well for governments, for the drug companies, for the psychiatrists who put people on drugs then give them more drugs for the side effects; and for the legions of psychologists, nurses, social workers, administrators and lawyers who keep this huge industry of alienation going. It also works very well for people who have troublesome relatives and prefer them sedated. It just doesn't work for the people it ought to work for.

Given all that we know about mental function (including the principles outlined above), mental disorder is not just a reality, it is wholly predictable. Because we can understand how people get trapped in distress, we can then work out how to assist them to regain control. That is, we can indeed have a non-physical science of mental disorder. The biocognitive model is a formal, non-reductionist *science* of mental disorder which starts with several premises:

1   Mental disorder is a reality;
2   It arises by predictable malfunctions in the emergent mind;
3   The mind can only be understood in its own terms, which are not those of the material universe;
4   We can apprehend those terms if we take the correct approach;
5   This allows us to see the processes by which people become mentally disordered and offers a rational process of treatment and recovery.

7.10 Sad or depressed?

We accept that the idea of "normal sadness" is not an oxymoron [4], yet most people accept that there are states of misery that go far beyond normal experience. For example, it sometimes happens that a desperately unhappy person starts to believe that his bowels have rotted and are poisoning his mind with toxins; or that he is such a bad person that he deserves to die; or that people who come in contact with him are defiled and need to die to be free of the contagion. The only way most people can understand these states is as illness, a physical malady starting in the brain. However, if we accept the dichotomy between sadness and illness, the immediate question is where to draw the line. That is, what is the demarcation criterion between normality and abnormality? Needless to say, nobody has ever found one. I say that's because there isn't one.

Biological psychiatrists say they just need to do some more research to find it. However, in the meantime, they need to be sure they aren't missing any cases. That is, if they are overlooking genuine cases of depression, then it will not be possible to find the point of demarcation. And from this point arises biological psychiatry's imperialist imperative: they must keep taking over more and more cases to ensure they haven't made a false negative diagnosis. Inevitably, as the field of psychiatric illness grows and grows to encompass more of what our grandparents thought was just a part of life, the field of normal sadness is whittled down until it disappears into the clinic.

Can this process be resisted? It can, but not with any reliability, just because the humanist and the reductionist camps speak totally different and, indeed, incompatible, languages. In a human-centred psychology, and given its context, a mood of intense sadness may be entirely normal. The biological reductionist model denies this just because it sees its assessments as context-free. By their definition, intense sadness is a symptom, and symptoms are biologically-determined, not context-driven. Therefore, all talk of "understanding" a person's misery is as meaningless as "understanding" his fever, or the pain of his broken leg. The only meaning to be understood is the patient's score on, say, the **Beck Depression Inventory** where a certain score *means* depression which *means* brain disorder which *means* treatment. And, of course, if the patient declines treatment, that proves he is even more in need of it, so he will be detained and given it.

The question then arises: Can mental states be considered as context-free episodes? In other words, can we divorce the fact of a mental state from its meaning? In the first place, it is not possible because all mental states are informational states, and there is no such thing as an informational state without meaning or context. Information without meaning equals noise: "The king took a walk today." Which king? Where? When? Why? Devoid of context, the statement cannot be used to create in the listener's mind a facsimile of the speaker's mental state so, as language, it fails. Ultimately, a mental symptom arises just because of its context; it is the context that determines why the subject experiences just this symptom and not another.

Thus armed, we are now in a position to begin the process of assembling what psychiatrists have long talked about but never but never delivered: a model of mental disorder that integrates the biology, psychology and sociology of human life.

References

[1] Luria AR (1980). *Higher cortical functions in man*. New York: Basic Books.

[2] Sapolski RM (2017). *Behave: The Biology of Humans at Our Best and Worst.* London: Bodley Head.

[3] Kahneman D (2011). *Thinking fast and slow.* New York: Allan Lane.

[4] Horwitz AV, Wakefield JC (2007). *The Loss of Sadness: how psychiatry transformed normal sorrow into Depressive Disorder.* New York: Oxford University Press.

8 Implementing dualism: the emerging model

I must freely confess, the difficulties and objections are terrific, but I cannot believe that a false theory would explain, as it seems to me it does explain, so many classes of facts.

Charles Darwin (1809–1882)

Psychiatry remains the discipline of medicine that has yet to grasp the nature of the disorders it treats. This explains why it lacks the power to resist social and political fads claiming to solve the problem of human mental distress.

Paul McHugh (b. 1931).

It is better to be wrong than to be vague.

Freeman Dyson (1923–2020)

8.1 Mapping the pathways

You have been invited to a typical university neuropsychology department in order to watch an electroencephalography experiment, aimed at mapping data flows within the brain. Through a two-way mirror, you watch as a student volunteer is brought into a quiet and dimly-lit room. The experimenter seats the student, called Ms A, in a comfortable chair facing a screen on the opposite wall and fits a special cap over her head. Connected to a computer by a loom of wires, it measures the electrical activity of the brain.

After making sure the apparatus is working, the tech places a device with two buttons under the student's right index finger and instructs her what to do: "Watch the screen. You will see photographs of buildings or landscapes from around the city, of five seconds each. We want to know whether they are familiar. If a picture is familiar, press the right hand button, if not, press the left. Keep this going until you are told to stop." Briefly, he watches the subject testing the button a few times, then gives a thumbs up and leaves the room. He can be seen through a window watching the display on a monitor.

Shortly, the researcher touches a keyboard and the screen in front of the subject displays a landscape. The subject's responses are shown on the bottom of

DOI: 10.4324/9781003183792-8

her screen and on the researcher's monitor. On the tenth change, a plain screen appears with some decorative marks, thus: หยุด. Five seconds later, the pictures begin again. The subject seems to hesitate a little, then continues pressing the button. After a further minute, the screen goes blank. The experimenter comes in, removes the buttons and the subject's cap, thanks her and indicates she can leave. The experimenter then brings in another subject, Mr B, seats him and repeats the procedure. However, when the tenth image appears on the screen, the subject stops pressing the button, sits back, arms folded, and waits. Shortly, the door opens and he is shown out, to be replaced by Mr C. Everything proceeds as before until the plain image appears. Mr C is perplexed and looks to the experimenter's window. He says something but the technician doesn't hear. As the pictures of buildings resume, Mr C repeats himself. Again, nothing happens. Mr C calls loudly, then shouts. Finally, he snatches the cap off and stamps out.

What can we conclude about the nature of mind from this experiment? The best place to start is the empirical facts. In the first part of the experiment, in each subject, the images evoked streams of impulses in the optic nerve which were conveyed back into the brain where they cascaded through a series of nuclei. At each junction along the pathway, the impulses were modified until they were projected to the cerebral cortex for final processing. The EEG then detected patterns of activity over the motor areas of the subject's brain, patterns which were almost identical for each subject and were causally related to movement of the hand.

However, when the new image หยุด appeared on the screen, the EEG tracings diverged. In each subject, activity in the visual areas in the occipital region of the brain persisted but in the first person, there was no detectable change in activity in the brain's motor area. The pattern associated with the rhythmic pressing of the button continued unchanged. In the second subject, activity in the motor areas ceased. The third subject showed similar activity to the first before he abruptly ended the experiment.

In each subject, the data flow from the picturess had two distinct mental effects, the immediate, ineffable experience of "something out there, on the screen," and the knowledge that the image was either novel or familiar. At this stage of our technology, the EEG is unable to detect the patterns associated with the different pictures. We simply have to accept that the subject "saw" each screen as different, and could correctly identify the various images displayed. Of courses, monkeys and birds, which know nothing about wavelengths, can be reliably trained to respond to different pictures so we can accept that there is a systematic or non-random basis to this process.

The interesting part of the experiment is when the symbols were displayed, because that is what they are, not just a pretty pattern. However, Ms A didn't "know" they were symbols in that they didn't evoke a familiar mental state so she didn't react to them ("took no notice"). This is the essence of language: an informational state is communicated from one entity to another through a medium by means of an agreed code. For us, language is simply a code which allows us to convey sets of instructions from one person to another on how to construct in the listener's mind a facsimile of the speaker's mental state.

For human communication, the message is selected by the speaker and conveyed to the audience with the intention that they will reproduce the speaker's mental state "either exactly or approximately,? as Shannon put it. This can only happen if speaker and audience use the same code to communicate. If, as speaker, you use a code that I know, then I will describe your utterances as having meaning, where "meaning" means "allows me to set up the particular mental state you intended." If I don't know your code or you don't use it correctly then, as in the experiment above, I will say your speech (or writing) is meaningless. Ms A was polite about it, Mr C wasn't.

Thus, at the beginning of the experiment, the technician had a clear idea in his mind what he wanted to convey to his subjects so he issued a set of instructions in the agreed code (English, as it happened). The subjects received the message as sound waves, decoded it, and recorded it as an instruction to be followed. None of that is conceptually difficult, machines do it all the time. Then, when the subjects saw the screens, they had to make a simple decision: Is this familiar or unfamiliar? The informational input from the retina that creates the experience of seeing the image also serves to generate a cognitive appraisal: "Seen it before or not." Because this item of knowledge and the experimental instructions are encoded in the same format, the cognitive item and the memorised instructions can then interact to produce an outcome, "familiar" or "new" (the sense of novelty is another internally-generated sensation).

In the next step, which is very fast and silent, this decision is conveyed to the motor area of the brain. The subject cannot introspect any part of this process, just as the workings of his liver are silent: the connections simply aren't there. Subsequently, each person's forefinger moved a number of times except in the case of Mr B after the symbols appeared, as he correctly interpreted them as an instruction to stop. Why did he do this? Because that's the instruction conveyed by the symbols in another code he has learned: Stop. In addition to English, Mr B speaks a language that uses a completely different alphabat, Thai. In Thai, หยุด (pronounced 'yut' to rhyme with the English 'put') is the agreed code for 'stop whatever you are doing.' In Figure 8.1, it appears in a familiar format:

However, Ms A and Mr C hadn't been exposed to that particular code and therefore weren't able to set up a facsimile of the experimenter's intention (his mental state) in their minds, so they kept pressing the button until the experiment came to an end.

It is clear that memory plays a very big part in this model, as it does in any model of information processing.[1] In any modality, the very concept of processing implies that some input flows through a fixed structure in order to effect changes which yield the desired output. In the case of the human brain-mind system, there are two components to the "fixed structure." The first is the very

---

1 This is almost a truism, as Turing showed. Without a form of memory to process a data flow, there is "mere transmission" of data, not processing. The instructions for processing are stored in memory.

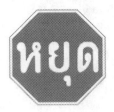

Figure 8.1

obvious microstructure of the brain itself. In particular, this model proposes that there are highly systematised logic gates coded into the cell walls of cerebral neurons such that any informational flow (in the form of neuronal impulses) cascades through them and is thereby coherently transformed.

The second component is the higher level store of instructions, or memory, which manipulates the systems of logic gates to produce different outputs. By this means, a finite number of physical logic gates can produce a potentially infinite output. However, this second level of "structure" is not quite so fixed as the first. While the logic gates are part of the structure of the neuronal wall, their function is determined by coded instructions in other sets of gates. That is, they can be switched on or off according to different inputs. In turn, they can influence the action of the memory stores, setting up a plastic and highly recursive data processing system, one which has no specified beginning and, short of death, no end.

Remember that while input states are added arithmetically, the complexity of the output states rises exponentially. The sense of self as an enduring entity arises from the complex interaction of a huge number of input and output states in different modalities, with the sense of continuity deriving from memory. As Turing expected, the model can account for all conceivable human behaviour but memory is critical: without memory, one's sense of being a specific human, or of dealing with another human, breaks down entirely.

8.2 Personality

This model is consonant with the fundamental structure of Turing's conceptual universal computing machine, i.e. an input tape, a read-write device which can access a store of memory, and an output tape. In essence, that reduces the human being to a set of core functions but it does not, of course, say anything about the actual structure of the computing machinery. Central to this model is the concept of a memory store. The example in Sect.8.1 relied on two basic features of human memory: the long-term, as in language, and the short-term, as in the instructions given by the experimenter. Subjects A and B followed the instructions like robots but Mr C didn't follow the rules. He showed the intrusion of a third set of coded instructions in that, when frustrated, he became irritable and impulsively broke the rules of the experiment. This type of behaviour is normally known as *personality*, character, temperament, or by a dozen other names. Everybody knows what it means but it isn't easy to define. Before we can continue, we need to specify it. The following section is based on material in Chapter 5 of [1].

The broadest possible *definition of personality* is this:

8.2.1 Personality is the universal set of interactions between the individual and his environment.

Immediately, we see some practical problems with this. For a start, it's encyclopaedic, you would need a very large computer to record all the details. Second, it wouldn't be finished until the person dies, which isn't much help. Third, it doesn't actually do what we want from a definition of personality. It's nice to know what a person has done in the past but what we really want is some idea of what he's likely to do in the future. That is, we're interested in his habitual modes of behaviour because we know from experience (induction) that whatever he's done in the past, he's likely to keep doing in the future. A person who has habitually turned up to work on time is likely to continue doing that. On the other hand, a person who rarely gets to work on time is more likely than not to be late tomorrow, and to show other areas of irresponsibility. Thus, we restrict our definition to read:

8.2.2 Personality is the set of habitual patterns of interaction between the individual and her environment.

This still doesn't tell us much because people change as they age. More importantly, under unusual or very difficult circumstances, they may behave in unexpected ways. So we arrive at this definition:

8.2.3 Personality is the set of habitual patterns of interaction between the individual and his environment, in the stable, adult mode of behaviour.

We're getting there but it's still very broad. We know that people who are sick, or who have had a knock on the head, or are intoxicated with any of a thousand substances will act strangely: out of character, we'd say. Our definition needs a further restriction:

8.2.4 Personality is the set of habitual patterns of interaction between the healthy, sober individual and her environment, in the stable adult mode of behaviour.

Because personality is really about what distinguishes us one from the other, we want to exclude the common elements of behaviour, such as language, culture and so on.

8.2.5 Personality is the uniquely distinguishing set of habitual patterns of interaction between the healthy, sober individual and his environment, in the stable adult mode of behaviour.

Now because these are habitual patterns, it is fair to assume that something is generating them. The model we are using is mentalist, just because, apart from saying it exists, physicalist (biological) models can't tell us anything interesting about personality. By continuing this process, we will arrive at the following definition:

8.2.6 Personality is the *total set* of explicit and implicit mental rules (including attitudes, beliefs, etc) that *generates* the uniquely distinguishing habitual patterns of interaction between the healthy, sober individual and her environment, in the stable adult mode of behaviour.

Personality *just is* a set of rules, just as grammar is a set of rules. That's why you can't see it or experience it in yourself. Where are these rules? In memory. Can we know them all? No, partly because there are too many, and partly because a lot of them were learned preverbally, or subverbally, as in a moment of agitation. Many more were simply absorbed in much the same way as we learn a language. The linguist, Noam Chomsky (b.1928), says that human children can extract the general rules of their language from exposure to just a small sample of the possible sentences in the language. They don't even know they have these rules but they are nonetheless real and effective.

This is also true of learning the myriad rules of behaviour, of our attitudes to ourselves and the world and our place in it. You could say that from very early in life, we are mining the environment (natural and social) for rule-like generalisations, using them to create our own mental lives. That is, the unique collection of rules, beliefs and attitudes, both explicit and implicit, that generates the distinguishing habitual patterns in my stable, healthy, sober adult mode of behaviour *just is* my personality. It's the framework on which my sense of self is built. Fleshed out with memory, emotion, goals, ambitions and current experience, I assemble a coherent sense of self. This is important, because under certain circumstances, such as very high arousal, the unified sense of self can start to break down, which is in itself terrifying to the subject.

Personality is no more than a set of rules that govern how I interact with the world, how I behave, how I feel, how I initiate actions and how I respond to everything around me. As a crude approximation, you could get away with calling it a program, or set of programs, and I wouldn't argue too strenuously but remember, it's unique. No two people on earth have exactly the same set of rules, that would be impossible. Similarly, nobody knows all the rules that govern his life, any more than he knows all the rules of language. Look at this pair of phrases:

A green great dragon.
A great green dragon.

Which one is correct, and why? Everybody older than about ten who speaks English knows that the first one is incorrect. Why? Because the order of adjectives in English says that size comes before colour (in fact, the order is opinion-size-age-shape-colour-origin-material-purpose. Hardly anybody knows this explicitly, but everybody can tell when the rule is broken. According to Mark Forsyth, who should know, the example comes from JRR Tolkien's first attempt to write a story, aged six).

This puts us in a good position to define personality order:

8.2.7 An ordered or *normal personality* is said to exist when the individual's set of rules is *both* internally coherent, thus generating a euthymic (pleasant) state, *and* consistent with the larger society's set of rules, thus leading to harmonious and productive interactions.

That makes sense: a pleasant personality is more or less what other pleasant people in that community at that time say it is. This leads us smoothly to a formal, *explanatory* definition of personality disorder:

8.2.8 *Personality disorder* exists when *either* the individual's set of rules is internally incoherent, thereby causing inner distress, *or* when it repeatedly brings him into conflict with the larger society, resulting in distress in the individual and/or society, *or both*.

Personality *just is* a set of rules which are coded into the brain's microstructure. Some are more or less fixed, others are less rigid. They act upon the data input to produce the output, and are in turn influenced by the input in an endless and vastly complex, self-reinforcing pattern. However, there are other, major governing influences in human behavior, which this model can incorporate.

8.3 Personality: traits and drives

When we talk about personality, we try to convey the broad impression of a person's behavior. Is he tidy or messy? confident or insecure? pleasant or abrasive? adventurous or resistant to change? sociable or solitary? Does he worry endlessly about his health or ignore it; is he fastidiously organised or wildly impulsive? Is he honest and rule-abiding or dishonest? Because there are so many rules involved, they form natural groups or clusters, generally known as traits. In fact, they aren't; traits are genetically-determined but early researchers were convinced personality is genetically-determined so the name stuck (that was in the days when it was thought the human genome contained about 3million genes; latest count is about 21,500, which is enough to convey the instructions for building a brain but not enough to encode all the information needed to set up a system of rules called personality). I prefer the term 'personality factors.' A personality factor is simply a cluster of rules, each of whose members are more like each other than they are like members of another cluster.

Depending on how the subject's behavioral rules are sorted and grouped, we can have as few as three major factors (Hans Eysenck: extraversion/introversion, psychoticism and neuroticism), or sixteen, as in Raymond Cattell's 16 Personality Factor model. Today, there is general agreement that there are five distinct, major factors which, together, can account for the complexity of human behavior. The five-factor model is usually known by the acronym *OCEAN*:

*O*penness: inventive/curious vs. consistent/cautious.
*C*onscientiousness: efficient/organized vs. easy-going/careless.
*E*xtraversion: outgoing/energetic vs. solitary/reserved.
*A*greeableness: friendly/compassionate vs. challenging/detached.
*N*euroticism: sensitive/nervous vs. secure/confident.

Because people can score low or high on any one of these five unrelated factors, that gives 2^5 or 32 sub-types. I don't believe this is anywhere near enough as it cannot convey the full impact of, say, a paranoid personality in its many variants. In addition, if there is a genetic factor in personality, this model does not provide any suggestion as to how it will be implemented by the physical brain. In order to do this, we need to step back a bit to avoid becoming bogged in detail.

When talking of the genesis of personality in any individual ("Why are you the person you are?"), there aren't many choices:

8.3.1 All personality is genetically determined (innate), or
8.3.2 All personality is acquired through early life experiences (learned), or
8.3.3 Personality is a combination of innate and acquired factors.

At this stage of our knowledge, only a fanatic would take either of options (1) or (2). For option (1), there isn't enough material in the genome to code for the complexity of personality. Relying on acquired rules is by far the more economical stratagem. For (2), the correlation between early life experiences and adult outcome is surprisingly inconsistent and unreliable. Option (3) is the moderate position but where do we start? Probably the most reliable starting point would be on Mars, seated among a group of Martian anthropologists who study the inhabitants of the third planet from their sun. Asked for their impression of humans, the first point they would make is that Earthlings are social creatures. That's true, we like to cluster together in tight-knit groups, to the extent of building giant cities where we can physically live on top of each other. Their second point would be that as soon as humans have formed a group, they arrange themselves in a dominance hierarchy. This is sometimes a democratic process but is more often accomplished by a great deal of pushing and shoving, even outright violence. The important point about it is that it never stops. "Uneasy sleeps the head that wears the crown," quotes one of the Martian scholars, to a round of chuckles.

And that leads to the next point our Martian anthropologists have noticed in their thousands of years of observation, our ceaseless violence. Unquestionably,

H. sapiens is the most wantonly violent creature on its home planet, so violent that their name for us translates as *Homo violentus.* Indeed, our neighbours worry that we may not survive our own violence. Granted, we like to play, but all too often play blurs across into violence; it is often difficult to tell where one stops and the other starts. Similarly, we like pretty things and we love to decorate ourselves, but often that means dressing ourselves in gorgeous military uniforms so we can invade our neighbors to loot and destroy their beautiful buildings, then we give each other more medals and ribbons to wear.

These are not fanciful comments but are very real. What we show is essentially the same nature as other higher primates, especially chimps and baboons. In brief, humans are in the grip of higher primate nature. We are social animals; we form tight-knit social groups in which we establish rigid dominance hierarchies, enforced by threatened or actual violence. We form close affectionate bonds with our kind but, at the same time, we are deeply mistrustful of "the other," for whom hostility is the default stance (xenophobia, fear of the stranger). We are highly territorial (possessive); yes, we like to play, we decorate ourselves and our territories, we have an aesthetic sense in most sensory modalities ... *but* our standard method of resolving any difference of opinion is by aggression. These features are universal, intense, and are readily visible in our close kin, the higher primates, so it is hard to avoid the suggestion that they have a strong basis in biology.

We could then make the case that, to a large extent, *the unique personality is essentially how the individual implements these biological imperatives, where differences in implementation are determined by early life experiences.* This leads to an interactive biological and psychosocial model which has the particular advantage of permitting personality change in adulthood. That is, if life experiences are such as to cause the subject's rules to change (sometimes for the better, more often for the worse), he becomes a different person without the change itself being a form of mental disorder.

Instead of having a welter of biological "drives," this model proposes that a very large part of our behaviour is governed by the single emotion of *anxiety:* in general, we avoid anything that increases anxiety and we do anything that reduces it. Being physically close to other humans reduces anxiety; separation increases it. We can imagine a strong evolutionary advantage in this feature as early hominids that remained close to their troop would be more likely to survive than those that wandered off alone, especially at night. The group is kept together by fear of separation. Separation anxiety is very real in infants, but persists into adulthood. People who choose to lead solitary lives, either because they experience little separation anxiety or because of high interpersonal anxiety, are deemed mentally disturbed (autism, Asperger's syndrome, schizoid or avoidant personality, etc). Now that doesn't make sense: why should there also be interpersonal anxiety? That leads to the second feature noted by the Martian anthropologists, our strong inclination to form dominance hierarchies.

In primates, *dominance* is about reproduction; there is no convincing reason to believe humans evolved differently, so we'll accept that and look at the details. As will be described in detail in Chapter 9, dominance is about feeling good, and feeling good is about hormones. Specifically, dominance is about testosterone: the dominant or alpha male struts around feeling good just because, and as a direct result of being on top, he is pumping out lots of testosterone. If we change the order, putting him at the bottom of the pile, his secretion of testosterone drops. Instead of being cock of the walk, he skulks at the edges of the group, quickly getting out of the way of the more dominant males, sulking, brooding, plotting miserably and living in fear of more trouble. This relates directly to the psychological perception of winning. Thus, a man who for any reason feels inferior will actively avoid competition, or even anything that will lead to competition, meaning contact with other people, just because he knows he is more likely to lose than win, and then things will get worse. Why does anybody in these democratic times feel inferior? The answer is the same today as it was in autocratic or anarchic times - physical strength, to compete with other men; physical appearance, to attract women; intellectual ability, to plan and keep in front; and, of course, what we will call self-esteem. We will come back to this but remember that all of this applies equally to women.

Dominance is a two-way process: the dominant dominate, and the dominated let them (or know better than to challenge them). Different people try to exert dominance by different means but there are innate advantages such as how first born sons achieve at a higher level than their younger siblings; tall people usually dominate smaller; and society favours the good-looking over the homely ("It's always tempting to impute unlikely moral virtue to the cute"). People who, for a variety of developmental reasons, feel anxious when challenged or threatened, are more likely to give in and avoid the challenge, leading to the schizoid or avoidant personality. The exception is when people flip the arousal of anxiety into the arousal of rage, and attack at the slightest hint of a challenge. This we call aggressive or antisocial personality disorder.

Because the majority of people spend the majority of their time low in the dominance hierarchy, there are a lot of anxious people around at any one time. Some people learn to channel their apprehension constructively, so they forge ahead while others find less productive or frankly maladaptive ways of dealing with their anxiety, and life gets worse. These include drugs and alcohol and anything that is now called compulsive or addictive behavior, such as gambling, promiscuity, compulsive work ('workaholic') or, these days, obsessive solitary pursuits such as on-line gaming, marathon running or body-building. Some people try to control their fear of impending trouble by imposing an oppressive order on their physical surroundings, such as obsessive cleaning or meticulous organising, while others try to control the human world by insisting everybody follow rules to the last letter.

Many people refuse to accept that they are anxious; instead, they blame everybody around them for their constant discomfort. This is the important group of paranoid personalities, one of the most important of which is the jealous personality. Rather than admit he may not be good enough to keep his girlfriend, a man starts to blame other people for trying to steal her from him, or to blame her for thinking of leaving him. Others live in a state of fear from not knowing what is likely to happen next, so they start looking for conspiracies. Some learn to use the law to bludgeon people into submission (vexatious litigants) or become obsessively involved in matters or right and wrong or justice; others dive into the supernatural world and are never seen again; and all of them are convinced the world is against them, that they are being held back by persecution and not by their personal inadequacy. At the core of the paranoid personality is a sense of self-righteousness, which conceals the void of negative self-esteem. If you have nothing better to do one day, you could look at some well-known politicians in terms of their personality disorders.

Some people give up trying to feel calm in ordinary society and opt out. In the old days, they could join a monastery or the Colonial Service but these days, there are motorcycle gangs, Goths and punks, anarchist and Trotskyite groups, as well as those hardy perennials, the military and police services. Stamping around in a uniform with a pistol on your hip conceals all sorts of personality in-adequacies (for more detail on this approach to personality disorder, see my monograph *Anxiety: The Inside Story* [1]).

Finally, it is essential to note that there is no such thing as a category of personality disorder. Normal personality blurs imperceptibly with abnormal on any parameter you mention, and you are free to devise your own. All you have to do is find a natural cluster of behaviour and attitudes and give it a name. Fear of illness? Hypochondriasis, so much more expressive than mere neuroticism in *OCEAN. Pathological jealousy*, also known as the *Othello syndrome*, is a very real thing; I don't think saying a man (or woman, it's nearly as common in women) scores low on Agreeability conveys quite the same sense of calculated menace.

All this is a wordy way of saying personality is built upon a fairly elementary genetic basis, a process in which a basic suite of innate tendencies is shaped by a myriad life experiences to produce the complexity we readily recognise in each other (but not in ourselves, of course: my personality is just fine).

Finally, if personality is what a group of people from a similar background don't have in common, then *culture* is what they do. For any group of people, culture is the set of shared or common behavioral rules but we want to exclude language, so we refine the definition thus:

> Culture is the set of shared, non-linguistic behavioral rules within a stable human social grouping.

The concept of culture is very broad, including such quintessentially human activities as religion, food, sport, politics, finance and industry, literature and the performing arts. We don't normally think of culture as a set of rules but it de-volves to just that. With religion and football clubs, for example, we probably prefer to say "I believe ...." but a belief is just a rule or proposition one is prepared to act on. There is, however, no fundamental or ontological difference between personality and culture. They are both clusters of rules which can be used to interact with a variety of inputs to produce a particular output.

Remember that because there are so many rules, and they are often contradictory, it isn't always clear which one will dominate at any particular time. Today, I may be feeling good and I put some money in a collection bowl on the basis that that is what one should do. Tomorrow, somebody may have upset me or I may have lost some money so I walk past the collection bowl, telling myself that people should look after themselves, or there are too many cats anyway. Because there are so many rules of conduct, we can usually justify our actions without too much effort.

8.4 Language and Dreyfus

"Because personality is really about what distinguishes us one from the other, we want to exclude the common elements of behaviour, such as language, culture and so on."

What is the relationship between personality and all the other sets of rules? Every human has a potentially infinite range of what we can call output states, or observable behavior, including language, culture (such as convention, religion, politics, sport, among others), occupation and so on. Each output state is the product of a set of rules which determines the behaviour. Rules controlling the output state known as *language* have their peculiarities but they are not unique: at base, they are just a set of standing instructions as to how to act (speak) given certain contingencies. Language rules give us the means to communicate with other humans (and animals, of course); they say nothing about what we will say.

There is nothing magic about language; it is just a shared set of rules that allows me to recreate in my mind just what you have in your mind – or the bit of your mind you want me to know about. Perhaps you ask me to give you *ein roter Apfel* or even แอปเปิ้ลแดง. That's fine as I know those particular codes, so an understanding of a red apple clicks into place in my private informational space (note that I didn't say an image clicks into place; we operate at much more subtle levels than that). If, however, you asked for красное яблоко, you'd go hungry as I don't know the code used by 150 million people in Russia.

This also works for dishonesty: if I don't want you to know what I've been doing, I deliberately use our agreed code to cause you to set up a completely different mental image. The philosopher Harry Frankfurt (b. 1929) defines a lie as:

> ...an act with a sharp focus .... designed to insert a particular falsehood at a specific point in a set or system of beliefs, in order to avoid the consequences of having that point occupied by the truth [2].

The liar, as he further explains, has two subsets to his mental state, the truth, and what he intends you to accept as the truth. He knows the truth but he doesn't want you to know it, or that he knows it differs from what he has conveyed to you. In order to achieve his goal of deceiving you, he must acquit two steps: to convey the falsehood to you, and then to hide from you the fact that he actually knows the truth. Because he controls what he tells you, you get one informational subset but not the other, so you set up just that mental state in your head: "Oh, you don't have any apples today? That's a pity."

The clear implication here is that we "think" (whatever that is) at a level below or removed from spoken language. Before I act, I don't need to "say" to myself, "Oh, that vase is teetering, I'd better grab it quickly," because it would be in bits by the time I'd said that mouthful. All that happens is that I see it and, in an instant, I act. In that instant, I compute a cluster of decisions to reach a single outcome:

> That is a glass vase;
> The vase is unstable;
> The vase is about to fall;
> If it falls it will be smashed;
> I don't want it to break;
> I need to move quickly;
> OK legs and arms, do your job.

All of this takes place extremely fast and entirely at a subverbal level. If people want to use the expression 'unconscious,' I won't argue (although I don't like its Freudian connotations). Obviously, if you want to continue the computational metaphor, there is a vast amount of work to be done in each of these decisions: How do we know it's glass, how do we know it's a vase, what do we know about the laws of gravity, the rules of value, how do we make any decision, how do we activate the musculature of arms and legs to jump up and catch the vase just before it falls? There is no robot even remotely conceived that can do that sort of thing in the time available.

This is what the philosopher and early critic of *artificial intelligence* (AI), Hubert Dreyfus (1929–2017) had in mind in his (pointedly polemical) treatise from 1972, *What Computers Can't Do* [3,4]. During the 1950s and 60s, AI researchers were making wild claims for their field, claims which annoyed Dreyfus, who had extensive training in continental philosophy and clear ideas on the concept of consciousness - well, very much clearer than the IT people, who were thinking at the level of high school students (i.e. the age when they stopped worrying about such ephemeral matters and took up the certainties of mathematics and engineering).

Dreyfus concluded that the conceptual direction of AI at the time was essentially doomed, that it could never achieve what its proponents claimed, and that the idea of machines matching human intelligence was a fool's errand. He based his argument on what he identified as four major assumptions which AI people took as axioms but which were, in fact, no better than hypothetical suppositions. He believed they needed to be examined and tested. If this were not done, the entire project was doomed to lose itself in endless dead-ends, like a man who wanted to get to the moon climbing a hill and telling his friends "Oh boy, I'm making real progress here." The assumptions he identified were named the biological, the psychological, the epistemological and the ontological.

Briefly, the *biological assumption* underlying IT at that stage was that the brain uses some sort of Boolean or similar algebra based in biological on/off switches. The *psychological assumption* said the mind could be viewed as a logic device operating on symbolic representations of items of information, according to formal rules. The *epistemological assumption* was that all human knowledge can be formalised into rule-abiding systems. Finally, the *ontological assumption* was that every fact in the universe can be represented in a symbolic system. Needless to say, the model developed so far in this book relies on exactly those assumptions except for one point: we are not talking about artificial intelligence.

His book generated a furore, leading to a huge secondary literature. Decades later, he felt that he had won the argument, although it was clear that AI had evolved away from the basis of his case - as we would expect in science. If we use a medical analogy, imagine that the surgeons who discovered anesthesia in 1846 decided that the world was their oyster, and they should be able to do cardiac transplants within ten years. Had they tried, their results would have been disastrous. They knew nothing about asepsis, fluid metabolism, artificial respiration or immunology. As the bodies were wheeled out, a skeptic would have felt on strong grounds to argue that major surgery was forever impossible.

In fact, it took 120 years before the ill-fated Louis Washkansky briefly woke with a stranger's heart. Every step forward generated two more questions that had to be answered by dogged research in hitherto-unforeseen fields, and the same thing has happened in AI. Everything was much, much more difficult than the early researchers imagined, but there has been progress. For example, something that Dreyfus specifically said would be impossible, rapid real-time machine facial identification of individuals, is now unfortunately commonplace. In big cities in China (and yes, all cities in China are big), if you jay-walk, you will be captured on CCTV. Within twenty seconds, you will be identified and a fine debited against your credit card, not to overlook the permanent black mark on your social record. Of course, the process uses a lot of computing power but that computational power runs software that was not conceived when Dreyfus wrote his book. Computing power is nice but, without the software, it's not much help.

Even though Dreyfus' argument was pitched against the possibility of machines ever doing what humans do effortlessly, his critique still has validity. In this model, of course, we're arguing backwards: can the machine analogy capture what humans do to the extent of providing insight into mental disorder, or are we forever doomed to regurgitating the mantra "chemical imbalance of the brain"? Central to his case was the notion, derived from continental philosophy, that human intelligence has a crucial, but largely unconscious, contextual element which can never, as AI demanded, be rendered explicit as formal rules. In the example of the falling vase, above, we have touched on the concept of contextuality or nested assumptions. We can look at his objections in turn.

First, the *biological assumption*, that the brain uses some sort of Boolean or similar algebra based in biological on/off switches. The biological on/off switches are a reality but there is a great deal more to brain function than that. Does it matter to this model whether the brain uses a Boolean-type algebra? No, not in the slightest. We don't know anything about brain codes but we are sure of one point: it uses something. Its exact nature is a matter of empirical research. For the biocognitive model, the question is: Can a Boolean system mimic brain function to the extent of advancing our understanding of mental disorder? My case is that it can, that it *models* brain function but it makes no claim as to the nature of the processes it models. As George Box observed, "All models are wrong but some are useful." As it happens, I think the brain does use a Boolean-type process, but that is an empirical matter.

Second, the *psychological assumption*: the mind can be viewed as a rule-based logic device operating on symbolic representations of items of information. At the outset, the biocognitive model states that this assumption is wrong. It is the case that the *brain* is a logic device, manipulating data flows according to rules coded into its physical structure to underwrite symbolic representations, but the mind itself is the emergent informational space generated by the brain. The mind is an entity with real powers but it is not a device.

Third, the *epistemological assumption*: all human knowledge can be formalised into rule-abiding systems. At different points in his book, Dreyfus argued that in order to implement a computational model, the brain would need vast memory capacity, far beyond anything conceived at the time he was writing. He should have paid closer attention to Moore's Law. In the fifty years since his work was first published, the number of transistors on a chip has doubled about twenty times, meaning 2^{20} more than when he was working. That is an exceedingly large number; it gives us the physical capacity to do just what he said was impossible, even though it has taken longer for the software to catch up. For better for worse, as governments and private companies implement the panopticon, that is now happening. But can *all* human knowledge be formalised into rule-abiding systems? The answer is yes, if it consists of information that can be communicated from one person to another, it can. The only information that can't be formalised is the ineffable information of our private experience, but that's a fairly boring truth so his objection loses a lot of its impact.

Four, the *ontological assumption*: every fact in the universe can be represented in a symbolic system. It is certainly the case that every material fact can be thus represented, but are there immaterial facts? The biocognitive model states that there are immaterial facts: seeing green is one of them, tasting an olive, or feeling a twinge of pain are others. But nothing hinges on those facts just because they are now and forever private: colours, flavours and pains exist only in the mental informational space of a suitably equipped entity. If the entity didn't see green as we understand it, but "saw" something else, or even tasted it, nothing would change. As long as it can reliably detect light at a frequency of 5.45×10^{14}Hz, its internal representation is, as we could say, immaterial.

Finally, his *contextual objection*: human intelligence has an unconscious contextual element which can never be rendered explicit. In fact, that objection is neutered every day: a large part of a psychotherapist's job consists of helping people render explicit the unconscious assumptions that have been controlling their lives. I suggest Dreyfus had spent too much time talking to continental philosophers and not enough talking to troubled people. However, unless we can show how the immaterial mind can influence the material body, he would still win his bet.

8.5 Bridging the gap

Rules mean nothing unless they can be instantiated or put into effect. The whole of this model hangs upon one critical point: showing how an insubstantial rule coded in an immaterial space, such as "Always close the door when I leave," can lead to physical doors being pushed shut. Conceptually, this is not difficult. In principle, the point of interaction of mind and body is the point at which a computational neuron makes contact with an effector or transmitter neuron. Mind and body interact at a synapse, the anatomical junction between two neurons, where the axon from a neuron which takes part in manipulating the data input makes functional contact with the dendrite of an effector neuron, meaning a neuron with no computational capacity. The distal or efferent neuron may be a motor neuron, that is, it takes instructions and transmits them to a muscle fibre, or it may be secretomotor, a neuron which, when activated by a specific input, secretes hormones or other chemicals which act upon distal tissues:

> *The junction between mind and body is the set of all junctions between afferent (input) transmitting neurons and computational neurons and, on the effector side, the computational neurons and efferent (output) transmitting neurons. There is not a single mind-body junction. Instead, there are billions of tiny input and output junctions, each transmitting a minuscule part of the total input or output state, and all devoid of mental properties.*

Recall this:

> "... the *brain* is a logic device, manipulating data flows, which themselves underwrite symbolic representations, according to rules coded into its physical structure, but the mind is the emergent informational space generated by the brain."

All mental activity, including decisions, is subserved by neuronal activity. As an input travels through the computational networks, it is modified until it reaches the end of the road, as it were, the last neuron in the network. But it doesn't just fade away, or go around for another loop, the data exits the computational system as an instruction, in order to act on neurons which themselves act upon the real world. On the afferent side, there is a a two-, three- or four-step process between the receptor neuron and the computational neurons of the cerebral cortex. On the efferent side, the process is reversed. From computational neuron to the outside world via the effector neurons is another two-, three- or four-step process.

The effector neuron is a bridge between the exclusively computational networks and the non-computational material body. At its input end, it can take signals from a computational neuron because it has the same input machinery as the computational neuron's output machinery. However, the effector neuron changes in mid-stream, as it were, because its distal end has a different output from a computational neuron. For example, a computational neuron (say in the frontal regions) cannot secrete testosterone, the essential sexual hormone. Instead, it sends instructions to a cluster of hypothalamic neurons to secrete a small peptide which then travels to the pituitary, causing the manufacture and release of a large hormone (follicle-stimulating hormone FSH) which travels via the blood to the testes. There, it acts on its target cells to stimulate them to produce and release the essential hormone testosterone. In principle, this is fairly simple but the details have taken nearly 80 years to specify.

Let's return to Richard Watson's definition of dualism, in Sect.1.2:

> The crux of dualism is an *apparently unbridgeable gap* between two incommensurable orders of being that must be reconciled if we wish to justify our assumption that the universe is comprehensible.

In the human, the two incommensurable orders of being we need to reconcile are the substantial or material body, and the insubstantial or immaterial mind. In fact, we can reconcile any incompatible systems, as long as we have the right connecting cord, one which can take instructions in one form at the input end, and emit them in another form output. As everybody knows these days, all we need is the right three pin plug. For humans and other animals with mental properties, the interposed neuron, bridging the gap between the computational network and the physiological body (Descartes' brute mechanism), is just that plug.

References

[1] McLaren N (2018). *Anxiety: The Inside Story*. Ann Arbor, MI: Future Psychiatry Press.

[2] Frankfurt H (1986). On Bullshit. *Raritan Quarterly Review* 6, No. 2 (Fall 1986).

[3] McLaren N (2012). *The Mind-Body Problem Explained: The Biocognitive Model for Psychiatry*. Ann Arbor, MI: Future Psychiatry Press.

[4] Dreyfus H (1972). *What Computers Can't Do: a critique of artificial reason*. New York: Harper and Row.

9 Applying the Biocognitive Model

Success is not enough. One's friends must also fail.

Gore Vidal (1925–2012).

...no one ever seizes power with the intention of relinquishing it. Power is not a means; it is an end. One does not establish a dictatorship in order to safeguard a revolution; one makes the revolution in order to establish the dictatorship. The object of persecution is persecution. The object of torture is torture. The object of power is power.

George Orwell (1903–1950), *1984*.

9.1 Male behaviour: the Challenge Hypothesis

Male behaviour, all the way from lizards and fish to dogs and humans, demonstrates striking similarities, mostly mediated by testosterone. For a detailed account of this very widespread hormone, see *The Challenge Hypothesis,* Chap 8 in [1], which gives all the citations for this chapter. Briefly, *testosterone* is required, not just for reproduction, but for assertive/aggressive behaviour. It is a powerful anabolic hormone with a wide range of effects, on the brain, muscle and other organs, and is very much a "feel good" hormone. High levels of testosterone are related to assertive, exploratory and dominant behaviour, while low levels lead to the opposite: submission, withdrawal and avoidance of social contact. An important point is that in order to do its job, testosterone must be secreted and available before it's actually needed.

Most animals have a clearly defined breeding season during which they show stereotyped behaviour. Outside this season, testosterone levels in adult males are at low ebb, enough to maintain the secondary sexual characteristics at basal level but not much more. Behaviorally, non-breeding males are fairly passive and disinterested. However, in response to specific environmental signals, such as temperature, daylight hours, rainfall, etc, the production of testosterone increases to a much higher level. In *birds*, in which this phenomenon was first noticed, the male develops gaudier plumage and starts to establish and defend a territory so he can attract a female. He acts aggressively toward other males and is

DOI: 10.4324/9781003183792-9

dominant toward females. Physiologically, the gonads enlarge and initiate spermatogenesis. This higher level is sufficient to lead to breeding but, in most species, if the male is challenged in his home territory, he shows a sudden, further surge of testosterone. This is important as the hormone is necessary to maintain the aggressive and dominant behaviour he needs to defend his territory and his mate. The more a *breeding male* is challenged, the higher his levels of testosterone. At the same time, the higher his levels, the more challenges he will perceive, and the more likely he will be to respond to challenges aggressively. Clearly, the cycle can become self-perpetuating.

In most animals, provocative triggers are very specific, especially the sight, sound or scent of another male. This is enough to provoke the defensive surge of testosterone which allows him to respond to the challenger, hence the name of this phenomenon, the Challenge Hypothesis [2]. The perception of a threat directly stimulates the hormone that is needed to confront the challenge; without just that surge, he will be unable to defend his territory and his family.

For every challenge, there can be only one winner. After a battle, testosterone levels in the victor will remain high, or some species show a further surge. In this state, he is more likely to perceive challenges or threats, and more likely to respond aggressively to them. The loser, however, goes into a decline. By the fact of losing, his testosterone level drops sharply, as does the aggressive and domineering behaviour that he showed leading up to the fight: animals know perfectly well when they have lost. The concept that the perception of a challenge provokes a surge of the hormone that is needed to respond to the challenge is fundamental to understanding male behaviour. Most emphatically, this applies to *Homo sapiens* [3].

In adult male *H sapiens*, testosterone levels are partly mediated by the sleep-waking cycle but also by a range of other events. The first, of course, is sexual stimulation, which leads to the surge of testosterone which is necessary for the individual to become aroused and sexually capable. If the hormone is blocked, say by drugs or intoxicants, he can't perform or won't last the distance. Second is the expectation or anticipation of sexual activity. In the main, Western men show higher levels of testosterone on Friday and Saturday than on Monday and Tuesday. The male partner of a couple who wish to become pregnant will show a testosterone surge on days 11–14 of his partner's menstrual cycle.

In addition to the central role of testosterone in reproduction, it is intimately tied to the *dominance-submission* axis in human affairs. High levels of this hormone feel good. Artificially boosting its levels causes the subject to feel more powerful, more capable, more adventurous and more inclined to explore further. He will try to dominate people in his surroundings either verbally or physically, and will be sexually more assertive with women. But the process goes two ways: the awareness of a challenger in the surroundings produces a surge of testosterone, which leads to assertive and dominant conduct. All too often, this provokes the other man to respond with self-assertion or aggression. This can quickly become a struggle driven by what we could call a testosterone arms race. Depending on the setting, including cultural mores, this may become a physical fight. After the competition resolves, the winner's testosterone levels will stay high; he will strut around, aggressively challenging men and acting in a sexually assertive manner toward women. The loser's hormone levels quickly decline and he will slink away, ashamed. As a brute fact of physiology, winning feels great, losing is miserable. That is why humans are so competitive, that single point explains a very large part of human behaviour, the worst part [4].

This applies to all challenges, not just sexual encounters. A man who is booked to play an important match at 2.00pm will start to show a rise in testosterone about midday. The bigger the competition, the earlier the surge starts. A debate will have the same effect, as will a court case (not only in the defendants but especially in the lawyers for both sides; only judges are immune because boredom is inhibitory), any challenging investigation, and so on. It can also be seen in men driving a big or powerful car or controlling any large machine, and, most dangerous of all, in handling weapons. Simply picking up and fondling a gun will produce a surge of testosterone, which is highly reinforcing. A man who has used a rifle even for target practice will feel good and will be more likely to want to do it again. And again [5].

This pattern generalises to all species and all forms of dominance, not just sexual. The dominant or alpha male has higher levels of the hormone, which feels much better than the low levels found in his insecure, submissive or downtrodden conspecifics. If the chief of a group loses his exalted position, his levels of hormone will drop, leading to a drop in his dominance behaviour, and to a dramatic reduction of his sense of well-being. Losers are more likely to be sick than winners. In humans, this pattern can be seen in any workplace, office, sports field, school, bar, prison or university, wherever men gather in groups. Above all, it is seen in armies.

It is almost impossible for human males to form groups without also forming a dominance hierarchy, just because being on top feels so much better than being on the bottom. This is quite separate from the usual reward of sexual success. Heterosexual men confined together, with no access to women, will still try to dominate each other but with little or no sense of primary sexual desire for each other. This was as true of the pampered court *eunuchs* of the Byzantine, Chinese and Ottoman empires, whose plotting and machinations were the stuff of legends, as it is of any army, prison, football club, pub, factory or office. It is also true of elderly men whose endogenous testosterone is low: being on top boosts what little hormone there is, losing reduces it.

Some people have tried to look at human behaviour as the outcome of a pleasure drive, or hedonism. Others see it as an expression of an aggressive drive but all of this misses a crucial point. The point is that dominating other people is inherently much more satisfying than being dominated, it feels better. Until we understood testosterone physiology, domination was just a brute fact of life, it's how we are. Over millennia, moralists have tried to tame these responses, telling men that winning isn't everything, that there's more to life than success, that there can also be a proud and valiant loser but who, even losers, believed that? Daily reality contradicted the moralists. As every male knows, as every human knows, winning feels so much better. This shifts the explanation of human aggression from the knowing or cognitive level, to an inaccessible and unreasoning level.

We can therefore see a very large part of human behaviour as the outcome of the hormonally-driven urge to dominate. Politics, sport, business, militarism of course, but even education and religion, are about dominance and control. Physical aggression is only one of many means by which people can come to dominate their neighbous. We don't dominate to get more sex, that's its reward; or to destroy, that's just letting them know who's boss; or to convert people to the true religion, religion is just another tool of the drive to dominate; or for any purpose that we can verbalise. We dominate to dominate, it is its own end: because of the testosterone cycle, it feels so much better to be on top:

> The object of power is power.

The drive to dominate, in women as in men, is absolutely fundamental to our concept of ourselves, to the extent that we hardly notice how strong it is, or how dangerous. We will look at the implications for a theory of mental disorder, but first, a little neurophysiology to settle the point articulated by Descartes:

> These questions presuppose amongst other things an explanation of the union between the soul and the body, which I have not yet dealt with at all (12 January 1646).

9.2 Mind-body interaction: testosterone

For a model of *mind-body interaction*, the crucial question is: How can thinking of an impending competition cause a surge in the one hormone that is necessary for success in the competition? Even though he knew nothing about hormones, Descartes intuitively understood the implications of this question. In modern terms, we would rephrase it as finding the relationship between a thought or idea and the gene expression needed to flood the bloodstream with a hormone. Is it true that, just by thinking, I can change my genes? The biocognitive model of mind says this is correct, that the thought content most definitely can and routinely does influence gene expression, but it goes further, by outlining the specific mechanisms involved.

The brain's various neurohumoral systems are of the same order as any other output state. That is, on the basis of a range of informational inputs, and operating outside the reach of introspection, the computational network makes very rapid decisions which activate specific effector systems. Needs are perceived by the same mechanisms as we perceive anything; decisions are made according to the body's perceived needs; and goal-directed actions are taken, in humans just as in other animals. In the simple case of deciding to lift one's right arm, it is a matter of connecting the computational neuronal system to a muscle by an efferent (motor) nerve, sending an impulse down the nerve, and up comes the arm. Granted, there's a little more to it than that but the principle is clear.

Other brain output systems are entirely physical with no cognitive input (in any sense of the term), e.g. the TRF-TSH-T4 feedback system controlling *thyroid* function. This type of system is wholly physical, a biological mechanism that is not joined to the computational network. Thus, it is closed to introspection or access by any sort of will or intent. The processes governing the body's thyroid status are entirely biological in the everyday use of the word, in that they continue to operate when a person is asleep or even in a vegetative state from brain damage. As far as we know, the brain's informational content, meaning its acquired knowledge, has no influence upon this system whatsoever. However, this is not true of the reproductive hormones, especially of testosterone, which is powerfully influenced by the subject's informational state, i.e. by what he is seeing and doing, and what he believes.

Unlike hormones such as thyroxine, testosterone in post-pubertal males is very much under cerebral control because the first elements in its production are neurons. Specifically, neurons in the hypothalamus which secrete *gonadotrophin-releasing hormone* (GnRH) are directly or indirectly under the active control of a number of different higher centers, including the prefrontal cortex, which is generally assumed to play a vital role in "executive decisions." From various sources, activating neural impulses arrive at the GnRH-secreting neurons in the preoptic and suprachiasmatic regions of the hypothalamus. From this point on, the system represents no conceptual problems.

In humans, the gene for GnRH, *GNRH1*, on chromosome 8, is activated to its expressive state by a specific pattern of neuronal impulses impinging on the neuronal cell body via a G-protein receptor chain. That pattern of impulse comes directly from the computational network, which is itself activated by a range of external and internal stimuli, including by the perception of a challenge. How do we know a challenge when we see one? There are two answers to this question. Firstly, I don't know, but I don't have to, because lyrebirds, lizards and lemurs are just as effective at recognising challenges as we are. Second, that's what sophisticated pattern recognition systems do, they make decisions, such as "Yes, this is a challenge." Using a range of inputs, a person can tell when he's being challenged or threatened, including the stance or tone of voice of the person in front of him, facial expressions, or simply by being ordered around. Even chickens can tell when they're being dominated.

Once activated, gene *GNRH1* immediately causes production of the decapeptide releasing factor, which travels via the secretory neuron to the pituitary portal system and thence to the anterior pituitary. There, stored luteinising hormone (LH) and follicle-stimulating hormone (FSH) are released into the bloodstream to travel to their target, the testicular Leydig cells. By a similar process of gene activation, testosterone is rapidly produced and secreted into the bloodstream, so that it can act upon its own target organs, one of which is the brain. The critical structure here is probably the amygdala, specific nuclei of which are active in aggressive behavior. All this takes place rapidly, less than a minute.

Using testosterone secretion as the case example, we have reached a solution of the mind-body problem. The generic principle is straightforward and applies at a myriad points in the CNS. The computational network reaches a decision and transmits a highly specific trigger to a particular or dedicated neuron receptor. This neuron can be either neurosecretory or part of the motor system, but the crucial point is that it does not make further contact with a computational neuron. Instead, by virtue of having differing forms of input and output, it bridges the gap between non-material mind and physical body. That is, it amounts to a solution to the problem that vexed Descartes four centuries ago, except this is hardly a novel solution.

Wherever we have two entities of incompatible form which interact, we need to explain just how they interact. Let's say we have two bodies, A and B, which, for some reason, can't interact. They could be two groups of people who speak different languages, or substances such as oil and water, or computers using different operating systems, or different physical machines, it doesn't matter; they can all interact if one condition is satisfied. For successful interaction, there must exist a bridging mechanism which can take the output of the first entity and convert it into the specific input of the second. If we want to mix oil and water, we take a long molecule which is neutral at one end and polar at the other. Because it is non-polar, the neutral end (usually CH_3-CH_2-) can dissolve in oil, i.e. it is lipophilic, whereas the polar end (usually -H_2-COO-) ionises in water and therefore attracts the highly polar water molecules. This specialised molecule, commonly known as *soap*, dissolves in neutral lipids at one end and polare water at the other, thereby forming a bridge between two immiscible substances.

Every day, in untold billions of machines around the world, a reciprocating output from one machine (usually an internal combustion engine) is converted into a rotary input for the next machine, such as a rotary drive shaft for a vehicle, cutter, crusher, plough etc. This is so elementary that we don't even notice it. By the same principle, a mechanical input from a steam or hydro turbine is converted into an electrical output by the specific means of a DC or AC generator. We can't hold a copper cable in a stream and expect to get electricity.

These are examples of one part of the physical world interacting with another part. We are also familiar with two informational realms interacting, such as two people who don't speak the same language. They need a third person to stand between them who can take the verbal output of one person and convert it to the verbal input of the second. This person, known as an *interpreter*, doesn't even need to know what the two groups are talking about to be able to do his job (although it helps). The concept of output information from one machine acting as the input for another is fundamental to our modern world. With computers, all we need is the connector plug and a driver program to convert the first machine's output into the input for the second machine. This fundamental principle is the nature of "...the union between the soul and the body..."

9.3 Hierarchies and dominance

Humans are hierarchical animals. Ultimately, the *raison d'être* of a *hierarchy* is not that it is efficient, or is aesthetically pleasing, or is democratic or meritocratic, or any such high-sounding talk. Instead, the entire motivation for this universal phenomenon is just that oppressing feels so much better than being oppressed. All the political, religious, economic and metaphysical justifications, the rationales and arguments, amount to nothing in the face of the brute physiological fact that a boss feels better than a worker, an effect mediated largely by testosterone. What about the palace eunuchs? In fact, they had endogenous testosterone from the adrenals but, being impotent, they also had lots of spare time to intrigue.

Everybody wants to be on top; all that counts is how one gets there. Some people rise in the hierarchy by honest hard work and self-denial, while others are granted high status by an accident of birth and need never lift a finger (which they soon regard as their birthright). Plenty of people accept they're not going far, and seem satisfied with a routine job and inoffensive hobbies, but they will still try to get to the top of the local sports club or school committee. Some try to slither up the ladder by cunning use of connections they have either been given at birth or have cultivated by stealth. Even people who are meek outside the home may well be tyrants as soon as the door closes but, all too often, hoping for protection, meek people marry a tyrant so they end up oppressed at work and at home. Some turn to crime as the only option for escaping a life of misery at the bottom of the pile but, within their gangs, they soon form an even more rigid and brutal hierarchy. Even the religious, who broadcast warm homilies on how everybody is equal in God's eye, form exclusive tribes with oppressive hierarchies based on the message that, because they are so humble, they alone will enjoy the Almighty's eternal largesse. Finally, some people declare war on the hierarchy. They may isolate themselves, so nobody stands over them, or try to bring it down so they can build their own, and the whole tedious process starts again.

Nobody should think that destructively competitive behaviour is something seen only in other people: we're all guilty. It may just be keeping up with the people next door, or shoppers jostling each other's trolleys, or drivers cutting each other off, thereby provoking the absurdly disproportionate and dangerous response called "road rage." It's needing to have the biggest child's party in the street, squabbling over who gets the corner office, worrying who has the latest phone or gadget, the coolest clothes or the hottest partner, the prettiest or smartest child, the showiest wedding or the biggest funeral. Some people show little overt interest in climbing the hierarchy because life has already convinced them it won't work and they will probably be worse off. These days, they can indulge their need to dominate by joining online games where, as virtual warriors, they are just as warlike and brutal as their brethren. There are no exceptions. A person who seems to have entirely opted out of the race to the top lives in a fantasy world where he is top dog in a hierarchy of one (even the expression 'top dog' says 'hierarchy').

In any hierarchy, there are always two views, the view from the top and the view from the bottom. Some people need to fight their way to the top because they want to dominate but there is only ever one throne in any kingdom, so a lot of people have to accept second best. Some of them are satisfied to be a courtier for life, while others who can't make that grade band together and resist any attempt to dominate them. The drive to dominate, and the drive to avoid being dominated, are opposite sides of the same hormonal coin. What is called *libertarianism* in its many variants is just a matter of avoiding the ignominy of low status by aggressively opposing any imposed limits:

> "Give me liberty or give me death."
> "You can take my gun when you prise it from my cold dead hands."
> "An Englishman's home is his castle."
> "All taxation is theft."
> "I can come into your restaurant without a mask if I like, you can't tell me what to do."

"You can't tell me what to do." Their fanatical hostility to government is based in the same hormonal drive as we see in baboons squabbling over females on the veldt. Of course, within their own bands, libertarians form hierarchies, just as the local bridge club does.

In the biocognitive model, human aggression (physical and verbal) is not a thing in itself, but is just one servant among many of the drive to dominate. Aggression is a tool of the urge to get to the top, while sex is one of the rewards, a fringe benefit but not the goal. People don't fight their way to the top in order to get more sex, they get to the top and then realise how their new-found status opens novel sexual vistas. Take away the sex and they won't give up their role. And judging by all the old men (and women) who are obsessed with power to the point of mania, the lust for power, the drive to win, long outlives the lust (and capacity) for sex as, from long experience on both counts, the novelist, Gore Vidal, knew:

> As one gets older, litigation replaces sex.

Litigation, of course, is all about winning. That's what it *is*. Young men may use physical aggression to get ahead, but old men, who are just as determined to win, rely on cunning and subterfuge, generally with much greater success (àAge and stealth will always overcome youthful vigour").

A very great deal of human behaviour is driven wholly by the urge to win and dominate [6]. It is not just outright competition, such as sport, of course, but vast swathes of activity are directed at scrambling to the top and then kicking away the ladder to stop any competition. Think politics, business, hierarchical religions (that's almost all of them), academia, show business and the fashion industry, gambling and, above all, militarism. Add to that the peripheral industries generated by controlling competition, such as police, investigative and custodial services, financial controls, tax evasion and then frank crime and it is clear that a very substantial proportion of human production is directly aimed at getting power and holding on to it. It is hard to estimate but perhaps 40% of human activity is directed solely at competitive, and thus non-productive, ends. That should be rephrased: 40% of male activity is wasted. Generally, women work productively in the home and fields and factories without needing to crush the mother in the next home or the worker at the next bench every minute of the day.

If we look at male behaviour through the lens of an insatiable need to dominate and control people, we get a different and very unflattering picture of human society. Granted, there are plenty of caring and dedicated men working hard to better the world, or their little part of it. There are lots of good fathers and husbands and brothers and sons, quietly going about their business keeping the society ticking over. But there are also a lot who have only one interest, forcing their way to the top, regardless of the cost to others. And, at our dire peril, they are the driving force in the world. Wars are not started by school teachers trying to explain calculus, or by farmers, or fishermen, or factory workers, or doctors or truck drivers. They are started by men who fail to see that what feels good for them is probably not good for the larger society. This is called the *projectionist fallacy*, the notion that what I believe or what is good for me is what you should believe or what should satisfy you. Unfortunately, leaders don't ask farmers or fishermen before they start wars, as the brutally honest Hermann Göring (1893–1946) sneered at his trial at Nuremberg in 1946:

> Why of course the people don't want war. Why should some poor schmuck on a farm want to risk his life in a war when the best he can get out of it is to come back to his farm in one piece? Naturally the common people don't want war: neither in Russia, nor in England, nor for that matter in Germany. But after all, it's the leaders of the country who determine the policy, and it's always a simple matter to drag the people along whether it's a democracy, a fascist dictatorship, or a parliament, or a communist dictatorship.

Politicians and generals, industrialists and financiers live in a febrile hothouse where they hear only their own opinions reflected back to them. Look at this nakedly supremacist quote and work out who it was (answer at end of chapter. Clue: his first name was not Adolf):

> The conclusion of his speech was a declaration of supremacy that sought to outdo the other candidate: "It's never, never, never, ever been a good bet to bet against our country," he shouted, going on to say, "We never bow. We never bend. We never kneel. We never yield. We own the finish line. That's who we are."

9.4 Social behaviour

Despite this, the bonds that tie are ultimately stronger. Before there can be dominance hierarchies within a society, there must be a society itself. After the basic survival drives of air, food, water and shelter are satisfied, the first move is to cluster in groups, the social drive. People tend to see this as a positive thing but, if so, it is very difficult to formulate a non-question-begging explanation. The simplest account of the very strong tendency of humans to form social groupings is just that being alone is frightening. After millions of years of evolution, we are, as it were, wired to become anxious if we can't hear and see and smell and touch other people. We can see the same phenomenon in rhesus monkeys. For obvious reasons, this tendency appears to be at its peak in childhood but it remains a potent force throughout adult life.

On a physiological level, we could postulate that those neural centres sub-serving anxiety are subject to a steady stream of activating stimuli which are specifically blocked by hormones or transmitters produced by human company. In the absence of company, the blockade ceases and anxiety quickly starts to intensify, the only relief being to move closer to other humans. This automates the notion of a social drive, thereby satisfying Johnson-Laird's imperative. However, it immediately runs into the practical difficulty of how we account for the very real problem of social phobia: how can one and the same person have both a fear of being alone *and* a fear of being in company? The answer to that is stated daily by those who are afflicted with social phobia in that, yes, they fear being alone but at the same time, they also fear not being accepted, because rejection means being alone - for all time. As they move away from company, their fear of being alone builds up until it forces them back but, as they approach company, it abates only to be replaced by a new and more immediate fear of being rejected, humiliated and expelled.

Herding or flocking animals show this. An insecure or inferior animal doesn't push its way into the centre of the group, it hangs around on the edge, nervously watching the alphas (male and female) and ready to run at the first sign of an-tagonism. They fear being alone but they also fear punishment; the anxiety remains the same but, depending on where they are standing, the cause changes. This is a classic *approach-avoidance* dilemma although humans usually phrase it in terms of *self-esteem*: "I hate myself so I expect others to hate me too, and drive me away. But if they drive me out of their group, that will confirm I'm hateful and my life will be even worse. I'd better just stay in my room and play fantasy games."

Intellectually, this is not difficult to grasp. We can often recast what seems like a positive drive in terms of the negation of its opposite. In this case, we have replaced the idea of a positive attraction to human company with the concept of company being the negation of a fear of separation, but what about drives such as self-decoration, territoriality, or fair play? Self-decoration, I suggest, is only part of the drive to be dominant, the best example being the military. Everything about a squad of soldiers in dress uniform radiates power and dominance, especially mounted troops like the British Guards or French Cuirassiers. And the higher the rank, the more gaudy and gorgeous the uniform, with generals dripping with braid and decorations. But that's only to impress because most of them are well and truly past their prime.

Territoriality is one of the most basic drives in the animal world. Birds, fish and crocodiles are strongly territorial; there is really no need to explain it in humans in terms other than those that would satisfy those species. What we can be sure of is that territoriality has nothing to do with rationality, reason, altruism or any of the other excuses that have been extended for brutally invading the neighbour's turf, with or without slaughtering or enslaving them. At least Hitler was honest: "We need Lebensraum; there is plenty of land in the east; we are superior beings; so we will invade them, slaughter half the inhabitants and enslave the rest." *Slavery*, of course, is the ultimate domination, although being a detained psychiatric patient in Australia isn't far behind it.

Again, the concept of dominance is deeply entrenched in the drive to grab as much as one can, the problem being that we don't know when to stop. Presumably, when selection pressures were applying early in our evolutionary history, there was no such thing as "enough." Therefore, our drive to grab more and more does not come with an Off switch. So we have reached the position where the richest twenty-six men in the world own as much wealth as the poorest 50%, or 3.7billion people. In the US, the three richest men, Bill Gates, Jeff Bezos and Warren Buffett, own as much wealth as the poorer half of the US population, or 160million people. That this is destabilising to the society does not occur to those at the top of the pile, whose sense of entitlement is directly proportional to their wealth.

The concept of *fairness* would appear to be one of our higher achievements. As every parent knows, it appears early in childhood in more or less its final form: "That's not fair, he got more than me." "That's not fair, she won't let me have a turn." Again, I suggest we can tie it to the drive to dominate, or its corollary, the drive to avoid being dominated. Everybody intuitively knows when they're losing, and the concept of fairness, which reaches its zenith in documents such as the United Nations Declaration of Human Rights, is designed to stop people taking "unfair" advantage of their neighbors. What is unfair advantage? Strictly speaking, any advantage can be seen as unfair, to the loser if not to the winner, which is why we legislate for equality and against discrimination. Why is legislation necessary on such a fine moral point? Because, almost inevitably, people at the top don't think they got there by taking advantage of people. Instead, they will say they got ahead by hard work and self-sacrifice. Secretly and occasionally openly, they firmly believe they deserve their status and are inalienably entitled to it:

> It is easy to stand atop a mountain of privilege, and tell those at the bottom of the mountain that privilege is irrelevant (Rachael Ball, Human Rights Law Center).

In much the same way as Freud tried to reduce everything to sex, at this stage, it appears that a great deal of characteristic human behaviour can be reduced to the drive to dominate. Is this reasonable? I believe it is, for two related reasons. The first is logical, better known as *Ockham's Razor*, which tells us that the number of explanatory entities must not be multiplied beyond the minimum that will do the job. In the past, writers have postulated a huge range of drives, impulses, instincts etc, to "explain" human behaviour but, of course, they explain nothing. They simply stick a name on the behaviour without explaining it: it is not possible to name an entity and define it in the same illocutionary act. Second, regardless of how many drives etc. we need to invent, we still have to give an account of them that does not beg the question they are attempting to answer. In human terms, this means the ultimate explanation of innate (primate) drives will be physiological. The real value of the concept of a single drive based in established physiology is that it is explanatory, not descriptive.

At this stage, we have only one proven physiological explanation for a class of behaviour, the Challenge Hypothesis. Nothing else is even remotely on the horizon but, fortunately, dominance in its many forms amounts to a very large class of behaviour. If we can use this to explain more complex behaviour, we are satisfying the requirements of both Bishop Ockham and Philip Johnston-Laird. A single drive, clearly understood and modified to fit different circumstances, is a better explanation of the variety and complexity of human behaviour than a cluster of unexplained, unrelated "drives." We can examine this from the point of view of that bastion of rationality, *Homo economicus*, the centerpiece of the market economy.

9.5 Polanyi's *Great Transformation*

In 1944, an expatriate Hungarian historian and economist, Karl Polanyi (1886–1964), published a long and complex case against the classic idea that human economic activity reduces to the workings of an efficient self-regulating market. The efficient market model says that, as a collection of rational actors acting on nothing more than price signals, an unregulated market will efficiently allocate resources to investment, production and distribution. Drawing on his prodigious historical scholarship, Polanyi argued that this model will not just fail, but will inevitably lead to the destruction of society itself:

> All types of societies are limited by economic factors. Nineteenth century (Western) civilization alone was economic in a different and distinctive sense, for it chose to base itself on a motive only rarely acknowledged as valid in the history of human societies, and certainly never before raised to the level of a justification of action and behaviour in everyday life, namely, gain. The self-regulating market system was uniquely derived from this principle [7]

As the prerequisite for a genuine *market economy*, he explained, everything must be rephrased in economic terms and allocated a cash value. Everything, without exception, from which derives the idea that the primary elements of any human society - land, labour and capital - are to be recast as commodities, just like food, water, fuel and raw materials. That is, the fundamental structural elements of society itself were isolated so they could be allocated a price and thence traded. Thus, they were turned into commodities but, he argued, that process was artificial (fictional, in his term). In a true market economy, society as we know it is taken apart, its elements allocated a price, and the whole thrown into the meat mincer of the "free market." While an unregulated market must result in the destruction of society, attempts to regulate it mean it is no longer free. Moreover, such attempts necessarily open the door to manipulation of the market and widespread corruption. The concept of a self-regulating market, he argued, is either destructive of the society that the market is intended to serve, or inherently contradictory.

Nowadays, the notion of a rational, self-regulating market is de rigueur among economists, whose quants have marginalised Polanyi's erudite work (you could argue that they were unable to allocate a cash value to it, so they put it in the worthless pile). Thus, Margaret Thatcher (1925–2013) had no qualms proclaiming: "There is no such thing as society." What she meant was that, if they had any weight at all, social rules were necessarily subordinate to economic rules, an idea Polanyi found abhorrent because it epitomises the value judgement that private gain trumps humanist ideals at all times.

What, you may ask, does this have to do with mental disorder? In fact, with the international economy already in its third free fall this century, Polanyi's work has a lot in common with the biocognitive model. The clue lies in his concept of the fictional commodification of labour, but explaining this point will require a slight digression.

A market economy is an economic system in which decisions regarding investment, production and distribution are guided solely by price signals generated by the forces of supply and demand. Ultimately, Polanyi said, that is why the control of the economic system by the market is of overwhelming consequence to the whole organization of society: it means no less than running society as an adjunct to the market. Instead of the economy being embedded in social relations, social relations are embedded in the economic system. In this topsy-turvy system, he said:

> Nothing must be allowed to inhibit the formation of markets... Neither must there be any interference with the adjustment of prices to changed market conditions—whether the prices are those of goods, labor, land, or money. Hence there must not only be markets for all elements of industry, but no measure or policy must be countenanced that would influence the action of these markets. Neither price, nor supply, nor demand must be fixed or regulated; only such policies and measures are in order which help to ensure the self-regulation of the market by *creating conditions* which make the market the only organizing power in the economic sphere [7, p72; emphasis added].

If, however, the conditions must be created, the clear implication is that the self-regulating market is not a natural phenomenon, but is just one of a range of social forms that has to be built and put in place. Now we run into a problem because if labour is just another commodity, then who will set its price? Who, that is, should "(create the) conditions which make the market the only organizing power in the economic sphere"? Should it be the workers who are selling their time, or should it be the people who are buying their labour to work the land, mines, boats or factories to produce saleable goods?

> But labor and land are no other than the human beings themselves of which every society consists, and the natural surroundings in which it exists. To include them in the market mechanism means to subordinate the *substance* of society itself to the laws of the market [7, p75; emphasis added].

If the workers decide on the price for their efforts, then the land and factory owners will not be happy, as controlling the cost of the inputs is critical to the success of their ventures. For *capitalism*, of course, success is everything. There is no goal other than gain: that's what capitalism means. Thus, the wealthy will always fight the workers for control of the price of their sweat. During the early Industrial Revolution in Britain, this took the form of the *Combination Acts* of 1799–1800, which criminalised workers forming groups (industrial unions) or withholding their labour (strikes). These acts were passed by Parliament, which was comprised only of hereditary landowners and owners of capital, the very people who were building the first factories and who needed cheap labour to maximise their profits. The Acts handed to the capitalist class untrammelled power to dictate to their workers the price of their labour, and penalised workers when they objected. Manifestly, this was the polar opposite of the unregulated or *laissez-faire* market.

As a result, workers were little better than serfs: the first shots in class warfare, as it is now pejoratively known, were fired by the owners of capital. But why control the price of labour? Because it is a production cost, and producers always want to control costs to maximise their return. Thus, the essence of a true market economy is that it must treat 97% of the working population as a commodity, as mindless automata. If the workers can think and object, or take time off for their funerals, festivals or football matches, the market economy breaks down.

The question then becomes: Who is the market? If workers are excluded from making market-based decisions, then all that's left is a small clique of the wealthy who are running the show for themselves. This is partly because there is nobody else for them to run it for, but mostly because that's what people in positions of power do. In a labour market, workers don't profit from the market, they *are* the market. They are the goods being bought and sold but they are not themselves buyers or sellers. The elite are not buying and selling workers for the benefit of workers, because that's not what a market does: in the pig market, farmers don't buy and sell pigs for the benefit of pigs. A market functions to trade commodities for the benefit of those who own or want to own commodities; the profit goes to them, not to the commodities.

As a commodity called labour, workers are ciphers, a dumb herd who can be shunted around the place to maximise profits, regardless of their wishes or needs. In the end, when their jobs can be done cheaper overseas, they are sacked, just as horses were sent to the knacker's yard when internal combustion engines replaced carts. This was precisely what Thatcher meant when she cruelly mocked the idea that workers had the sentience to form a genuine society of human beings or, if they did, that it would amount to anything. To her and her privileged coterie, workers were just another commodity, and commodities must be controlled, not coddled. Imagine giving pigs a vote on whether they should go to the slaughterhouse.

By preventing workers having any say over the price of their labour, capitalism stripped them of their membership in human society, creating an underclass with no say over their destiny. However, and herein lies the rub, because according to the Challenge Hypothesis, humans don't like being treated as underdogs. In fact, they will fight to the bitter end to prevent it, as in Czarist Russia, Nationalist China, the American colonies, and so many other countries. So, in order to forestall more Bolshevik revolutions, workers had to be given certain rights, such as forming trade unions, the right to vote and then to form their own political parties. Giving workers the vote? That meant the newly-minted class warfare simply moved to a different level: union-busters and scab labour, gerrymandering, deregistering voters, and suborning workers' political parties.

The most sophisticated means of neutering the workers' political power was consumerism, the idea that capitalism would lead to utopia and everybody would be happy, so only a fool - or an anarchist - could object to the unregulated market. As Aneurin Bevan commented acerbically: "The whole art of Conservative politics in the 20th century is being deployed to enable wealth to persuade poverty to use its political freedom to keep wealth in power." But, Polanyi argued, built into asocial consumerism are two fatal flaws. Firstly, elevating endless selfish consumption to the level of the *raison d'être* of human life results in moral nihilism, including drug and alcohol epidemics, gambling and family breakdown (c.f. Aldous Huxley's notion of "pleasuring ourselves to death"). Second, unrestrained consumerism must destroy the natural environment because, as Kenneth Boulding pointed out, "Anybody who believes that exponential growth can go on forever in a finite world is either a madman or an economist."

Common sense dictates that the rational solution would be for the owners of capital to cede to the underclass a portion of their wealth, enough to make everybody happy. That, of course, will never happen: the Challenge Hypothesis says that those at the peak of the hierarchy will never willingly surrender their power. Using different arguments, Polanyi concluded that by stripping workers of their sense of autonomy, a full market economy contains within itself the seeds of its own destruction. As, from its own internal contradictions, with no communist threat to blame, the modern globalised market economy starts to collapse yet again, we can see why there is so much anguish and social restlessness today, and why the market economy can never rectify it. It all goes back to Ockham's Razor: The real value of the concept of a single drive based in established physiology is that it is explanatory, not descriptive. In the depths of the Second World War, Polanyi understood this intuitively.

9.6 The object of power

To return to Orwell's dystopian quote, the object of power is power. Humans dominate each other for the simple reason that being on top is so much more fun than being an underling. The lust for power doesn't need to be questioned because the answer is self-evident: it *feels* better, and now we know why. But the reason is dumb, it is mindless physiology, mere chemicals, equally at home in bull crocodiles in the mating season as in full professors in an elite university or politicians vying for the highest office in the land. The drive to dominate is innate, unreasoning, unthinking; it is a raw given or brute fact that the dominant person never questions, just because anything that feels so good can't possibly be wrong. Domination is its own explanation. All the justification and rationalisation, such as searching for weapons of mass destruction or bringing God or democracy to the downtrodden masses, is window dressing. At base, we are brutal, domineering creatures with a febrile lust for power second to none, as in this quote:

> The conclusion of Joe Biden's speech, as Hillary Clinton stood nodding in approval, was a declaration of American supremacy that sought to outdo Trump. "It's never, never, never, ever been a good bet to bet against the United States of America!" he shouted, going on to say, "We never bow. We never bend. We never kneel. We never yield. We own the finish line. That's who we are. We are America!"

Powered by the mindless ecstasy of a testosterone-fueled lust to dominate, the delighted crowd roared its approval, the only problem being that the other candidate in his red MAGA hat outdid them. While this wild, unreasoning excitement leads to war, the mindless destruction of war is absolute disproof of the idea that humans are rational economic actors. The innate drive to dominate results in the endless wars and dreadful social inequality that characterise modern human society. Unless we bring it under control, our species, if not the entire biosphere, is probably doomed. But the first step to bringing anything under control is to understand it. The biocognitive model offers a valid, non-question-begging explanation of that quintessentially human behavior, aggression. As a scientific theory of the mind, the biocognitive model treats it as an automaton.

References

[1] McLaren N 2012. *The Mind-Body Problem Explained: The Biocognitive Model for Psychiatry*. Ann Arbor, MI: Future Psychiatry Press.

[2] Archer J (2004). Testosterone and human aggression: an evaluation of the Challenge Hypothesis. *Neurosci Biobehav Rev* 30: 319–345

[3] McAndrew FT (2009). The interacting roles of testosterone and challenges to status in human male aggression. *Aggression Violent Behav.* 14: 330–335.

[4] Liening SH, Josephs RA (2010). It is not just about testosterone: physiological mediators and moderators of testosterone's behavioral effects. *Soc Pers Psych Compass* 3:1–13, 10.1111/j.1751-9004.2010.00316.x

[5] Klinesmith J, Kasser T, McAndrew FT (2006). Guns, testosterone, and aggression: An experimental test of a mediational hypothesis. *Psychol Sci* 17: 568–571.

[6] Mehta PH, Josephs RA (2006). Testosterone change after losing predicts the decision to compete again. *Horm. Behav.* 50: 684–692. http://www.ncbi.nlm.nih.gov/pubmed/16928375.

[7] Polanyi K (1944). *The Great Transformation: the political and economic origins of our time.* Boston: Beacon Press. Second edition: 2001, with a foreward by Joseph Stiglitz.

10 Psychopathology

I remember at an early period of my own life showing to a man of high reputation as a teacher some matters which I happened to have observed. And I was very much struck and grieved to find that, while all the facts lay equally clear before him, only those that squared with his previous theories seemed to affect his organs of vision.

Joseph Lister, Ist Baron (1827–1912)

I spent 13yrs at NIMH really pushing on the neuroscience and genetics of mental disorders, and when I look back on that, I realise that while I think I succeeded at getting lots of really cool papers published by cool scientists at fairly large costs - I think $20billion - I don't think we moved the needle in reducing suicide, reducing hospitalisations, improving recovery for the tens of millions of people who have mental illness.

Thomas Insel (b. 1951; Director, NIMH 2002-15)

Nothing could be more profoundly and meticulously deliberate than the measured footsteps of a man who no longer knows where he is going, though he is on his way.

Thorsten Veblen (1857–1929)

10.1 Reality of mental disorder

The central thesis of modern concepts of mental disorder is that every mental disturbance is but the surface reflection of an underlying biological disturbance of the brain. Unstated but central to the American *DSM* project is the idea that, for every separate category of mental disorder, there will be a separate and distinct, genetically-determined biological disorder of the brain, causing what is commonly known as a *"chemical imbalance."* It would follow, then, that for each mental disorder, there should ultimately be a separate and distinct drug treatment to correct the imbalance. We can call this a linear model of mental disorder, one which is entirely consistent with the formerly dominant concept of causation in science: A leads to B, which causes C, which results in D. Given any point in this chain of causation, its antecedents and postcedents can readily be determined. This is part of the rationalist mindset which gave us the Newtonian

DOI: 10.4324/9781003183792-10

model of physics, the classical model of economics, the germ theory of general medicine, evolution as a direct line from apes to the pinnacle of creation (we white males, of course), Marxist historiography and so on.

Trouble is, after decades of research and vast sums of money, not a single chemical imbalance has ever been found. One would think that this ought to give pause to the frenetic "search for the schizococcus," as the concept was once mockingly named, but no, not a word of it. Failure isn't in the lexicon of its devotees; for them, failure to find anything means only that it is elusive, not an illusion, that they must spend more money and more time until, one fine day, they will succeed. Be patient, and keep sending money.

In scientific terms, this is an absurdity. The search for what has morphed into the schizophrenogenic abnormal neural circuit is a fantasy that is driven by, and leads to, attempts to treat a non-physical matter by physical means [1,2]. At best, this is wasteful but, at worst, wantonly destructive (think lobotomies). This is especially true when most of the people at the receiving end of the treatment have not given informed consent, not least because, if they were given any information at all, it ranged from callously misleading to criminally culpable.

On the other hand, the biocognitive model is avowedly non-linear in intent. In generic terms, it is a *complex adaptive system*, meaning any system in which individually simple components or agents (in the case of the brain, neurons), controlled by a few simple rules and operating without central control, can produce complex outcomes which cannot be predicted from a full knowledge of the agents themselves (i.e. emergent phenomena, see **S.5.2**). It follows then that even small perturbations in the agents can produce self-reinforcing disturbances, eventually resulting in chaotic breakdown of the system, as measured by its outcome. The biocognitive model holds that firstly, mental disorder is a reality. Second, all behavioral disturbances produced by a physical brain disorder or disease can be duplicated by some change or other in the rules, but not vice versa: the set of behavioral disturbances produced by impairments of the rules greatly exceeds those produced by brain damage. Third, physical damage results in categorical or stereotyped disturbances, while mental disorder is distributed dimensionally, so there is no pure physical disturbance which can exclusively reproduce a syndrome of mental disorder.

In the great majority of cases, the brain of a mentally-troubled person is perfectly healthy, doing exactly what millions of years of evolution have shaped it to do. In this chapter, using the biocognitive framework as developed, we will outline a research program for some of the major psychiatric syndromes. Bearing in mind that there never was a formal linear model of mental disorder, it was no more than fervent hope masquerading as a scientific research program, the question this chapter will answer is: Can a non-linear model of mental disorder achieve more than the old linear approach?

10.2 Anxiety

At the end of the last chapter, I argued against the endless proliferation of un-proveable entities in any attempt at explanation. I will do the same here: in diametric opposition to the modern trend in psychiatry to find ever-larger swarms of ever-smaller diagnostic categories, I will show that, to a very large extent, there is only one underlying fault in mental disorder. That is, while a person may show half a dozen surface "diagnoses," there is only one underlying condition or "fault." In biological terms, that "fault" is not a fault at all but is simply the brain doing its job according to instructions sent to it by the mind.

In explaining mental disorder under Bishop Ockham's watchful eye, we need to find a single, pervasive mental element which is capable of causing widespread instability in mental function. The idea is that, directly or indirectly, that element alone can and does lead to impairments of mental function in its different facets (cognitive, affective, perceptual and effective). As will be clear from earlier chapters, there is only one non-pathological element which can broadly interfere with mental function, producing diffuse but real mental impairment. That element is, of course, the concept of *arousal.*

Physiological arousal is central to any concept of mental function, regardless of its ontology. Arousal is the mental difference between nodding off drowsily after lunch, versus jumping up and listening closely for what seemed like a strange sound. In each case, the brain is in a different and characteristic state but we, as owners of brains, don't know that. All we know is that we *feel* different. Being drowsy is not the same as the alert awareness we feel while waiting for the result of an important examination or interview.

As described in Sect.7.4, there is an important relationship between the level of arousal and the capacity to perform a task. At low levels of arousal (drowsiness), performance on any measure is impaired; same applies at excessively high level. In between, there is an optimal level of arousal at which performance is at a peak. This relationship is shown in the classic *Yerkes-Dodson curve* (See Fig 7.1). From the psychiatric point of view, it is the higher levels that count, but it is not just arousal *per se*, because people can be happy and aroused at the same time, and will often seek this effect. Instead, it is non-pleasurable arousal, otherwise known as anxiety, that does the damage.

The key to understanding mental disorder lies in reconceptualising the role of anxiety as the critical destabilising element in mental life. Anxiety is defined as the response to the perception of a threat, giving the *"fight or flight"* reaction. In daily experience, anxiety increases until the subject does whatever is necessary to alleviate the threat. That sounds all very sensible but the problem with anxiety is that it is the only recursive human emotion, hence its psychiatric significance. That is, it is the only emotion that, just by its presence, can act back to intensify itself. This is not a "fault" in any sense of the word, it is anxiety doing what it is supposed to do, alert the bearer to the presence of a threat and compel him to act on it. But if the threat is anxiety itself, then the subject is caught in a vicious circle of self-reinforcing, and therefore ever-increasing, agitation - with no upper limit. This is how a normal human reaction becomes self-destructive.

In terms of its unlimited capacity to interfere with mental life, anxiety is far and away the most powerful of all human emotions. Physically, it affects the body from top to bottom, from piloerection of the hair on the scalp, to sweating of the soles of the feet, and every system between. This is not surprising, as the role of anxiety is to save your skin. It alerts you to threats and gets you ready to deal with them, either by standing and slogging it out, or by running. However, as anxiety rises to the level of panic, it becomes counter-productive in that it so disturbs the individual's mental and physical function that it prevents a coordinated response to the threat. That is, the emotional reaction to the threat blocks an adequate response to the threat, thereby increasing the sense of danger. No other emotion has the same effect. This is the key to understanding the role of anxiety in producing diverse mental disorders.

There are several aspects to the anxiety response which must be clarified in order to understand what is happening to the individual (I'll call him a patient, because that defines the role). First, there is the somatic response, which consists of restlessness, shaking and sweating, racing or irregular heartbeat, churning stomach and nausea, and shortness of breath. The patient complains of a dry mouth, tightness or a sense of a lump in the throat (*globus hystericus*, which shows it's not a new idea), quavering voice, stammering or stumbling over speech, weakness, and dizziness, light-headedness or clumsiness. Different people show a variety of other symptoms, which may include numbness and tingling in the extremities, twitches and spasms, urinary urgency, bowel rushes, ringing noises in the ears, blurred vision or spots before the eyes, and so on. Because there is a great deal of overlap, it is essential for the psychiatrist to take a careful history in order to distinguish between somatic symptoms caused by anxiety and those due to more ominous physical conditions.

Second, anxiety produces characteristic cognitive effects. The most common is a sense of too many thoughts crowding into the head, producing confusion and uncertainty. In the main, these are thoughts of tasks that need to be done urgently to prevent trouble or other things that may go wrong, but they can be concerned with past mistakes or humiliations, or just the patient's endless failings as he perceives them. Some people complain that, when anxious, their minds go completely blank so they don't know what to do. Concentration and memory are affected early in the anxiety response. This makes it difficult to focus on tasks, leading to mistakes, which produce more anxiety, then more mistakes, in a self-reinforcing cycle.

There are also perceptual effects such as feeling trapped and needing to escape, or "the walls closing in." People commonly say that during an anxiety attack, they have the sense that the world looks different, or that they feel different, either from themselves or from others. They may have the impression of hearing things from far away, or looking down a tunnel at the world, quite often at themselves. These effects, traditionally known as derealisation and depersonalisation, are often attributed to something called "dissociation" but they are classic anxiety symptoms and do not imply any other process or condition.

Finally, there is the core of anxiety, the pure emotion of fear, the sense of impending doom or feeling of dread or terror that something terrible is about to happen. This is what converts the physiological arousal into something to be avoided or, for those who have experienced a bad attack, something to be feared in itself. A highly excited person will show much the same performance deficiency as an anxious person but they're having a good time and don't want it to stop. An anxiety attack is not good fun; it continues just because the patient fears his own anxiety and knows from experience it won't stop easily, if at all. But in itself, that belief is a scary idea, which is what keeps driving the anxiety and stops it fading.

It must be understood that there is only one sort of anxiety, the scary sort. All the current categories of diagnosis of anxiety are not about the anxiety itself but are concerned with the fairly limited number of options available to control it. My monograph, *Anxiety: The Inside Story* [3] looks at this in more detail but some of the options are:

Option 1. Patient can't control his anxiety, it rapidly intensifies and refuses to go away. Depending on what is more prominent, he will get a diagnosis of Panic Disorder or Generalised Anxiety Disorder. There is no real difference.

Option 2. Avoid anything scary. Leads to Avoidant Personality Disorder, Phobic Disorder, Social Phobia, etc.

Option 3. Use chemicals to control the fear, most commonly alcohol, which is the most specific, effective and dangerous of all anti-anxiety drugs, but also opiates, stimulants ("I feel ten foot tall and bullet-proof"), cannabis, benzodiazepines, antidepressants, antipsychotics, anticonvulsants, anaesthetic agents such as ketamine, and all other psychoactive or hallucinogenic drugs.

Option 4. Engage in some form of distracting behavior: Obsessive-Compulsive Disorder or Personality Disorder; and anything (wrongly) termed an "addiction," such as gambling, promiscuity, crime, religiosity, esoteric or mystical philosophy, physical exercise, dieting, eating, self-harm, and on-line gaming. Worry about health or follow food fads etc. Hypochondriasis.

Option 5. Try to take control of everything in the environment and react aggressively if anybody objects: variously known as Personality Disorder, or government (and yes, it is a tautology).

In the Biocognitive Model, the essence of the anxiety state is that the person is trapped in a self-reinforcing cycle in which slight anxiety causes some sort of physiological or psychological symptom which, in itself, the sufferer finds terrifying. This immediately intensifies the anxiety, producing more symptoms and more terror, as in this little interchange with a middle-aged woman:

Patient: My doctor keeps telling me I'm depressed but I don't think I am. She gives me these tablets but they don't work.

Dr: That's an antidepressant. You're certainly not happy but that's not the same as true depression, so those tablets won't work. Your real problem is anxiety.

Patient: Anxiety? Oh no, that's terrifying.

The recursive element is clear: anxiety goes from the mind to the body and then back again, in a self-reinforcing loop. This is true of any phobia:

Patient: I know it's silly, I know they can't hurt me, but I'm absolutely terrified of frogs.

Dr: No, you're not scared of frogs at all.

Patient: Oh yes I am, I know terror when I feel it.

Dr: No, you're actually scared of how you will feel when you go near a frog, and that's a totally different thing.

Social phobia is no different:

Patient: I have to give a talk at work but I can't do it, I'll have to resign.

Dr: No, don't do that, let's try to sort it out. What are you really scared of?

Patient: I'm scared I'll shake and sweat and stutter and make a fool of myself. Once, I even wet myself. I couldn't go through that again.

Dr: So you're actually scared of what they'll think of you? But look at it this way. You're scared you'll shake and sweat and stutter, but you only shake and sweat and stutter when you're scared. Do you see the vicious circle?

This is extremely common. Unfortunately, mainstream psychiatry has long failed to take anxiety seriously. Anxious people are routinely dismissed as "the worried well" and given short shrift. However, in a remarkable feat of marketing, drug companies have managed to convince regulatory authorities and general practitioners the world over that the correct, indeed, the *only*, way to deal with anxiety is to prescribe... antidepressants. Any less is neglect. That may be reasonable if antidepressants were effective and had no side effects but neither of those is true.

What is now happening throughout the western world is that anxious people, who are at least 15% of the population, are given drugs which are inherently destabilising to the brain, have a huge range of dangerous and/or undesirable side effects, *and* are highly addictive. And expensive. However, nobody is allowed to say they are addictive. If a patient takes them and then decides to stop, he will certainly experience unpleasant effects but he will not be told he is experiencing drug withdrawal. Instead, he will be told his original illness is returning and he must immediately resume his drugs, and probably take more. If the first lot don't work, new drugs are simply added until we reach the state where people are taking up to nine or ten separate psychoactive substances and everybody is wondering why they don't get better. Which leads to the next topic.

10.3 Bipolar disorder

In 1974, *bipolar disorder* was rare; so rare, in fact, that it didn't exist. In those unsophisticated times, it was still known as manic-depressive psychosis. It affected something like 0.1–0.2% of the population, meaning one or two per thousand. However, because they went in and out of hospital so often, they accounted for a much higher proportion of admissions than their incidence would suggest. This is because people diagnosed with schizophrenia went in but, quite often, didn't go out again. Added to that, the concept of "*rapid-cycling bipolar disorder*" certainly didn't exist.

On January 4th, 1976, I started work as a training medical officer at Graylands Mental Hospital, in Perth, Western Australia. I took over about forty in-patients and had to get to know them fairly quickly. One man, aged in his thirties, who was well-known in the hospital, had been admitted over the Christmas break, only three weeks after he had been discharged following a two month admission. The diagnosis was manic-depressive psychosis and, according to the case notes, he had been floridly psychotic when he was first admitted in October. After a week or two on his second admission, he seemed settled so I arranged his discharge. Three weeks later, he was back, agitated and irritable, demanding admission. Hardly had he settled than he urgently requested to be discharged. His wife had gone away for a few weeks but he became agitated without her, so he requested admission. However, he revealed she had told him that if he ever went back to hospital, she would leave him. As soon as he had settled, he was discharged and he later collected her from the airport as though nothing had happened. He was seen regularly throughout the year but did not require readmission.

However, his bed was hardly cold after his third discharge when I received a letter from the office of the director of Mental Health Services wanting to know why the patient had been discharged three times in barely seven weeks. Reading between the lines, I detected the question: "Do you know what you're doing?" I replied: The first discharge in early December had nothing to do with me, also true of his second admission at Christmas. The second discharge, in early January, was my decision that he was ready for discharge, and the reasons were covered in the case notes. The third admission came about because he had panicked when his wife went interstate to see her family (it later emerged that he was seriously jealous, which was based in intense personal insecurity), and the third discharge was as described, to get him out before she found out. What is the point of this little story? The point is that rapid admissions and discharges of people with what is now called rapid-cycling bipolar disorder were then so rare that it attracted official attention.

The next point, as mentioned above, is that in 1976, the syndrome was rare. However, it didn't stay rare for long. In 1980, the American *DSM-III* was published, which renamed it as bipolar disorder and dramatically loosened the diagnostic criteria. In 1984, Nancy Andreasen (b. 1938), former editor of the *American Journal of Psychiatry* and recipient of the National Medal of Science, said the incidence of bipolar disorder was 1% of the population, meaning it had jumped by 500–1000% in a few years [4]. By 2005, it was considered to be about 5%; by 2011, about 10.5% and the most recent figure I have seen came from Hong Kong, where it was estimated to be 15% of the population. That is, it has gone from one in a thousand, to one hundred and fifty per thousand population.

Now this is a little surprising. Normally, genetic disorders (as bipolar disorder is assumed to be) don't increase by 15,000% in one generation. So we have two questions to consider, its explosive increase, and the appearance of a new variant called rapid cycling. For mainstream psychiatrists, there is no problem: "We are now much better at diagnosing this disorder than in in the past," they will say, "and we have powerful new forms of treatment at our disposal." *But...* does that not suggest something? In general medicine, if we give a form of treatment but the problem gets worse and worse, we have to consider two possibilities for our failure. The first is that the diagnosis is wrong, and the second is that the treatment is wrong. On the medical wards, that response to treatment failure would be considered so basic as to be beyond comment. Unfortunately, psychiatrists don't see it that way. They do not believe their diagnosis is ever wrong, indeed, can *ever* be wrong, and they are wedded to their drug and other physical treatments, just because they have no other. If your only tool is a hammer, then everything looks as though it needs a nail.

The case against mainstream psychiatry is clear [5,6]. In the first place, the diagnostic criteria were loosened so far that anybody who complains of being "a bit up" and later "a bit down" will get the diagnosis of bipolar disorder. However, there is a very large group of people who have lots of ups and downs without actually being psychotic, those with anxiety disorders (including anxious personality, which the *DSM* system doesn't accept), and those with personality disorders. Two problems arise. In the first place, psychiatrists are not trained to assess personality, not least because they don't have a model of personality or of personality disorder. Second, they can't treat personality disorder. Their drugs don't work, and they are no longer trained in psychotherapy. Thus, a large proportion of people who get to see psychiatrists, usually because of a crisis in life, should be told to go home and see a psychologist *but...* Public psychiatrists are terrified of sending somebody home in case something goes wrong and they are held liable, while private psychiatrists don't like sending patients away because that's not how they make money.

Thus, the very large group of people with primary personality disorders are being rediagnosed with a mental illness, which means they can legitimately be treated with drugs. If they object, as people with personality disorders are wont to do, they can be detained, not on the basis that they are a danger to self or others, but on the basis that they have "unreasonably refused treatment." That way, they can be treated against their will. This accounts for the explosive growth of the diagnosis - well, this plus the sloppy diagnostic criteria that would allow a ham sandwich to be diagnosed as bipolar.

It is almost unknown for a person to be given the diagnosis of bipolar disorder and not be given a pile of drugs, and so we come to the second reason why this diagnosis has become the flavour of the century: the drugs. Psychiatric drugs are not chocolate drops. Without exception, they are powerful psychoactive chemicals with a very broad range of effects on the brain. While it is often said that they are specific to one neurotransmitter or another, there is absolutely no truth in this type of claim. All it means is that the drug company has tested the drug against one or two neurotransmitters (in rats) but not the rest of them. How many endogenous neuroactive chemicals are there? Well in excess of one hundred, and most of them can be either excitatory or inhibitory, depending on where they are. Despite all the high-sounding medical jargon, nobody has a clue what the drugs are doing at 99% of those sites. That is partly because they've never been tested, but also because nobody knows the relationship between neurotransmitters and mental function anyway.

The second factor leading to the explosive increase in this diagnosis is that psychoactive drugs work at or around the synapse, inducing changes which can be very persistent. However, the brain doesn't like this and constantly tries to restore its balance, fighting to correct the effects of the drugs by creating further changes in its chemistry. This is experienced as numbing, detachment and a variety of other unpleasant effects, so people usually complain. In turn, this leads, not to a reduction in dosage but to an increase, then more drugs, then more. If the drug is then stopped abruptly, it is like trying to drive with the handbrake engaged and then suddenly releasing it: the car shoots forward. This is what happens in humans taking psychoactive drugs, except we call it withdrawal from an addictive substance. Psychiatrists don't like the idea that their drugs are addictive, and have given the withdrawal effect the precious title "*discontinuation syndrome.*" Not only that, but Dr Google comes replete with seriously misleading information, such as:

Q: Does discontinuation syndrome go away?

A: With discontinuation syndrome, the symptoms eventually go away, usually within one to three weeks, but if you're having a relapse of your depression or anxiety, the symptoms don't go away and may even get worse.

This is completely false. This type of information is actually planted by drug companies, directly or via "astroturf" groups (groups which seem to be "grassroots" organisations but which are established and funded from above by drug companies). The truth is that withdrawal effects from psychiatric drugs *routinely* last up to two years and can be seriously disabling, up to and including psychotic episodes, with or without suicidal and/or homicidal impulses and actions.

From the point of view of the industries involved, this is a remarkable business model. Take a large number of people who are mildly dysfunctional for reasons of personality; tell them they have a serious mental disorder, thereby worrying them to the point they become increasingly dysfunctional; then give them drugs which, by universal consent, do nothing for the primary personality disorder but which are both inherently destabilising and highly addictive. By this means, a diagnosis can increase 15,000% in one generation, to the enormous profit of the psychiatric and pharmaceutical industries.

The modern trend leading to wild overdiagnosis and treatment of bipolar disorder is directly the result of sloppy diagnostic criteria; the inability of modern psychiatrists to take a proper history; their lack of proper models of mental disorder and personality disorder; their deskilling in the art of psychotherapy; and the actions of drug companies in pushing highly addictive and dangerous psychoactive chemicals on a gullible population (as in the *opiate crisis* in the US [7]). I do not doubt that, as a profession, psychiatry will have ample cause to regret this. The patients already do.

10.4 Depression

Depression is now regarded as having the highest *burden of disease* of all conditions. Again, we see the phenomenon of more treatment leading to worse outcomes. In the UK, 16% of the adult population take antidepressants; in the US, it is 13% and, unusually, Australia is a bit of a laggard, at only 12%. But that's not for lack of trying: in 1991, the figure here was just 1%. This explosive increase in prescription rates is built on the notion that depression is, in some critical sense, a pathological disturbance of physical brain function. The most common expression heard is "a chemical imbalance of the brain," a spectacularly meaningless shibboleth that is daily fed to the general public in a myriad ways. Beside enriching drug companies and causing an epidemic of obesity and impotence, what does this achieve? What, indeed, does it say about the formulation of depression as a "biological disease of the brain"? There is a growing awareness that there is something seriously wrong with the entire approach.

What we call depression is indistinguishable from grief, the biologically-determined reaction to the perception of a loss. Why this happens, we don't know as it is lost in the mists of evolutionary time, but the disease called depression is steadily encroaching on the life event called *grief*. It is, however, the case that the criteria for a psychiatric diagnosis of depression have been serially relaxed over the past forty years. It is also the case that, in most countries, a diagnosis of depression almost invariably leads to drug treatment. Very often, indeed, people don't even have to be depressed to be given the drugs. Anybody who complains too much is highly likely to walk out with a prescription for antidepressants. 40% of patients who are given them stop them in the first few weeks or months, either because of unpleasant to disabling side effects, or because they don't work. The remaining 60% of patients will become addicted to these very powerful, unpleasant and dangerous drugs. It is now common to see patients who have been taking antidepressants 25 or 30 years. *But...* they don't get better. That's *why* they take them decade after decade.

At present, we don't give antidepressants to grieving people so why do we give them to unhappy people with no obvious loss? That's the point: there is no obvious loss, so the same clinical phenomena are given a different name, from which automatically follows "treatment." It is a truism to say we don't know what triggers depression. If we did, we would call it a grief reaction, not depression. Nonetheless, by far the most common cause of unexplained or recurrent depression is an unrecognised anxiety state. There are several reasons why the anxiety is unrecognised. Firstly, since most people see anxiety as a moral failing, not as a recursive cognitive trap, sufferers often do their best to conceal it. Among the religious, anxiety is all too often dismissed as "lack of faith." This causes further distress to the sufferers who can't see how their faith is weaker or any less pure, but who are crushed into silence because they can't respond.

Second, most anxiety states are unrecognised because nobody bothers to ask the right questions. Finally, their significance is not recognised because psychiatrists think anxiety is trivial, a matter of "the worried well," not a life-threatening, crippling mental state with a high death rate which lies at the core of most mental disorder.

Being severely anxious destroys all pleasure in life. Try as they will, anxious people simply cannot break through the walls of fear which surround them. Gradually, they give up on activities until one day, they realise there is nothing left. The devastation produced by the awareness that they have lost everything with no prospect of life improving, that nobody understands and nobody can help, takes them to the brink. At that point, they experience total loss, they are forced to give up on life itself and sink into a profound despair. We call that depression but it is really the grief which comes from losing hope of ever being able to lead a normal life. Thus it is that people decide they may as well end their torture early. After the funeral, nobody can understand why it happened [8]: "He was such a happy person, he was polite and friendly and helpful, why did this have to happen?" No, he could act happy, but that was all.

From the medical point of view, being able to reverse the blockade of the "pleasure circuits" would be very helpful. However, that would require specific chemicals to target the receptors on a range of brain subsystems, about which we know nothing. Based on long experience, this seems most unlikely to be successful, not least because there are probably so many of them but also because the brain would fight to overcome the drugs used to alleviate the blockade. The biocognitive model indicates that the most successful way of reversing depression would be to stop sending signals of loss from the cortex to the deeper structures. In the case of depression resulting from unrecognised anxiety, this is relatively easy. All we have to do is give the sufferer some sense that:

a   his anxiety condition is not a moral failing,
b   anxiety can be dramatically improved, and
c   as a result, he will be able to lead a more fulfilling life.

The sense that there is a future stops the barrage of inhibitory signals generated a myriad times each day by his bitter awareness of his loss of a worthwhile life. Slowly, he will start to experience pleasure again. But, and this is the crucial point, the overwhelming majority of people complaining of depression do not require antidepressants. Giving antidepressants to unhappy people is like trying to blow the smoke out of a house without worrying about the fire. They need their anxiety states recognised and treated, then they feel better and, *mirabile dictu*, the "depression" melts away of its own accord. Nothing could be simpler. However, this formulation threatens the cosy and immensely lucrative duopoly of psychiatry and drug companies, so it doesn't get much air time.

10.5 Conclusion

The Biocognitive Model for psychiatry represents a total break with the past. It is highly-developed, far-reaching in its scope, firmly based in well-established principles from other fields of science, and leads to dramatically different ways of seeing old problems. More to the point, it says: Practically everything we are doing in psychiatry today is wrong, if not frankly destructive. It offers a new model of treatment that shifts the focus from blind meddling with the brain's function, to seeing humans as information-users with the capacity to get caught in self-sustaining mental traps. However, it also says we are dangerously irrational, which must be taken seriously. While this may be shocking to some, we ignore it at our peril.

References

[1] McLaren N. (2011). Cells, circuits and syndromes. A critique of the NIMH Research Domain Criteria project. *Ethical Human Psychology and Psychiatry* 13: 229–236.

[2] McLaren N (2013). Psychiatry as Ideology. *Ethical Human Psychology and Psychiatry* 15: 7–18.

[3] McLaren N (2018). *Anxiety: The Inside Story*. Ann Arbor, MI: Future Psychiatry Press.

[4] Andreasen N (1984). *The Broken Brain. The biological revolution in psychiatry*. New York: Harper and Row.

[5] Whitaker R (2009). *Anatomy of an Epidemic: Magic Bullets, Psychiatric Drugs and the Astonishing Rise of Mental Illness in America*. New York: Random House.

[6] McLaren N (2012). Chapters 14-16 of *The Mind-Body Problem Explained: The Biocognitive Model for Psychiatry*. Ann Arbor, MI: Future Psychiatry Press.

[7] Vashishtha D, Mittal ML, Werb D (May 2017). The North American opioid epidemic: current challenges and a call for treatment as prevention. *J Harm Reduction* 14 (1): 7. doi:10.1186/s12954-017-0135-4

[8] Senior J (2020). Happiness won't save you (commentary, *New York Times*). https://www.nytimes.com/2020/11/24/opinion/happiness-depression-suicide-psychology.html Accessed Dec4th 2020.

Part III
Conclusions

11 Pointing to the Future of Psychiatry.

I cannot accept your canon that we are to judge Pope and King unlike other men, with a favourable presumption that they did no wrong. If there is any presumption, it is the other way, against the holders of power, increasing as the power increases. Historic responsibility has to make up for the want of legal responsibility. Power tends to corrupt, and absolute power corrupts absolutely. Great men are almost always bad men, even when they exercise influence and not authority: still more when you superadd the tendency or certainty of corruption by full authority. There is no worse heresy than the fact that the office sanctifies the holder of it .... And remember, where you have a concentration of power in a few hands, all too frequently, men with the mentality of gangsters get control.

John Emerich Edward Dalberg-Acton, 1st Baron Acton (1834–1902)

Of all tyrannies, a tyranny sincerely exercised for the good of its victims may be the most oppressive. It may be better to live under robber barons than under omnipotent moral busybodies. The robber baron's cruelty may sometimes sleep, his cupidity may at some point be satiated; but those who torment us for our own good will torment us without end for they do so with the approval of their own conscience. They may be more likely to go to Heaven yet at the same time likelier to make a Hell of earth. Their very kindness stings with intolerable insult. To be 'cured' against one's will and cured of states which we may not regard as disease is to be put on a level with those who have not yet reached the age of reason or those who never will; to be classed with infants, imbeciles, and domestic animals. But to be punished, however severely, because we have deserved it, because we 'ought to have known better', is to be treated as a human person made in God's image.

Clive Staples Lewis (1898–1963)

I have felt it myself. The glitter of nuclear weapons. It is irresistible if you come to them as a scientist. To feel it's there in your hands, to release this energy that fuels the stars, to let it do your bidding. To perform these miracles, to lift a million tons of rock into the sky. It is something that gives people an illusion of illimitable power, and it is, in some ways, responsible for all our troubles — this,

DOI: 10.4324/9781003183792-11

what you might call technical arrogance, that overcomes people when they see
what they can do with their minds.

Freeman Dyson (1923–2020)

11.1 Computation and mysterianism

In this final chapter, I will look at some of the implications of what, via its approach to mental disorder, points to a radical reappraisal of the human condition. First, I want to reiterate that yes, this is a *dualist, computational model of mind*. There are several reasons for this, chief among which is that the evidence offers no other options. However, the term "computation" is left deliberately vague. For example, when whales create a "bubble net" to catch a school of anchovies; when a gannet plunges from 50metres high to catch a fish deep underwater, in the process correcting for refraction; or a mountain goat scampers down a cliff face while escaping a predator, there is some *non-conscious* inner process that amounts to a process of calculation. If we were to mimic it, we would cast in computational form, but we need to treat this carefully. Whether whale, bird and goat brains compute, in its strict sense, is an empirical matter that doesn't concern us because what we are trying to do is build a model of that process. I believe that, in some essential sense, they do compute but to reprise George Box's quote on the frontispiece:

> The most that can be expected from any model is that it can supply a useful
> approximation to reality: All models are wrong; some models are useful.

It is perfectly feasible that this computational model of mind is totally wrong but, at this stage, it does what it sets out to do. That is, it gives us a "useful approximation to (the) reality" of mental disorder, with far-reaching predictive power.

A similar objection is that it simply uses the modish concept of information processing rather than devise something new. Indeed, and that's what models do but, as concepts change, so too do the models. There is no point in returning to, say, Freud's hydrodynamic model or Clark Hull's electromechanical model. If anybody can improve on computation, I'd be pleased to see it.

On the other side lies the philosophical movement called *mysterianism*, which says we can never understand our minds just because our brains aren't up to it. That is a valid stance but it is very much an empirical claim, not metaphysical, and could be refuted tomorrow. The problems for mysterians are that a) they are venturing outside their primary field with no qualifications and b) making any predictions, especially regarding future technology, is always risky (see the fate of Dreyfus' predictions on facial recognition in Sect. 8.4). Meantime, they should take care not to fall into the projectionist fallacy, of believing that the limits of their own imaginations are the natural limits of the world. Still, insofar as mysterians limit themselves to finding fault with other people's theories, they have a valuable role.

11.2 Animal sentience

The next point concerns our relationship with our fellow earthlings. There are those who insist that all animals are "mere mechanisms" which require no understanding beyond physiology, and no consideration beyond satisfying our needs. It is, however, a fact that mammalian and other nervous systems, both central and peripheral, have far more in common than they have differences. For example, in their original work on conductivity in nerve fibres, Alan Hodgkin and Alan Huxley (1952) used the nerves of the giant squid, so our commonality extends back a very long way. Therefore, the burden of proving that animals have no sentience, or cannot communicate, or cannot realise what an abattoir is about, rests with those who insist animals are "mere brutes," just perambulated lumps of meat waiting to be skinned and eaten.

To me, it is the grossest conceit to say that the great apes - or even the little ones, - elephants, cattle and pigs and, above all, cetaceans and other marine mammals, are incapable of apprehending the world and their place in it in a way that has more in common with our own mental lives than there are differences. This compels us to reconsider our relationship with animals and to ask why humans, at all times and under all circumstances, have all the rights while cohabitants of our planet have none. As Mao Zedung said, "Power grows out of the barrel of a gun," and humans have all the guns.

11.3 Domination and our future

Domination is everything. A very large part of human behaviour is driven solely by the urge to dominate and control everybody and everything in range, a relentless battle for power. We can't put two people in a room together without a tussle to see who will dominate and who must submit. If we put groups of men together, the first thing they do is organise a friendly competition but, in no time, it can get out of control. Competitions, of course, have winners and losers, and winners soon start to think that they deserve whatever they have gained - and more. Winners never believe they have been lucky. Everything we do is based on the urge to push ourselves up the hierarchy, mostly by standing on the heads of those below and aided by kicking their feet out from under them. As soon as we start to get up the structure, we push away the ladder we have used to make sure nobody else can compete. In the battle for power, scruples are a handicap. It could be said that this drive, and others like it, are the reason why we have the concept of morals, since being fair and reasonable doesn't come naturally.

Everything is a battle for control and domination, from spectators roaring for their team, to superpowers building vast arsenals of *nuclear weapons*. The ultimate domination, of course, is slavery, the absurd idea that one person can actually "own" another. But what is owning anyway? All it says is: "I have put my mark on this, meaning I can do what I like to it but you can't do anything to stop me. If you try, I will bring all available force to prevent you, and the state will support me." If we "own" a piece of land, or a horse, or a child, or a slave, we don't somehow change its nature just by signing the contract of sale. As an indication, consider the idea of owning a cat: you may be able to put it to death but you don't own it. Nobody owns cats. All it does is give us certain power to exert "my rights" over yours. That's what domination is.

Over and over we are told the battle is between political left and political right, or Catholic against Protestant, or Christian against Muslim, or white against black, on and on, when the real battle is between those who want to dominate and those who aren't interested. In fact, the deception is even more basic, at the level of a small number of power-hungry people convincing the great majority that it is in their interest to leave their farms and factories, to submit to regimentation and wallop whoever the small group want them to. But, when the job is done, the regimentation doesn't go away.

Racism, sexism, colonialism, "ageism," all of these are just the concept of domination in different forms. Racism says: The colour of my skin says I can dominate you, I can tell you what to do; where to walk or sit; what jobs you can have; whether you will be politely cautioned or brutally arrested and beaten; the quality of your education and what you can learn; where your illnesses will be treated and where you will be buried. Racism just *is* domination, writ in coloured letters. Domination is men telling women what to wear, be it the burqa or working topless in a bar; it is female genital mutilation; it is telling people who they must marry, or who they may not; it is murdering people who marry the wrong person; it is denying the vote, gerrymandering, ballot-stuffing, and Big Money voting or politicians on company pay-rolls; it is teachers caning boys but not girls or girls being denied an education; it is child soldiers in Liberia, apartheid in South Africa and in the Middle East; a million Uighars in "reeducation camps" in Xinjiang, on and on.

Politics, sport, business, education, finance, religion, housing, fashion, clothing, cars, all is driven by the blind compulsion to build dominance hierarchies, to grab the power to get more of the biggest and latest in order to gloat and lord it over our neighbours. Sixty years ago, CEOs of American corporations earned, on average, twenty times the median salary of their employees. Now they pull in over three hundred and eighty times as much. Why? What do they now do that they weren't doing back then? Or what can they possibly do with all that money? They can't take it with them: as has been said, hearses don't come with towbars for U-Haul trailers. If asked, the only answer they ever give is "Well, that's the going rate, that's what others get so I should get it, too." What that means is "I don't want any of those bastards looking down on me, I can't handle the humiliation. So long as I can dominate the conversation at dinner parties, my workers can go hungry."

There is nothing inherently wrong with competition, it brings benefits, but the problem is we have no idea when to stop, and people get hurt. Initially, US President Harry Truman (1884–1972) said the US would only need about 200 hundred nuclear weapons in order to maintain a Pax Americana. At its peak, it had something like 29,000 nuclear weapons (and still has over 6,000). Nuclear powers built enough weapons to vaporise every square metre of the planet three times over, or the equivalent of 3.5 tons of TNT per person. They had to keep building them so they wouldn't feel the other side had an advantage over them. Meantime, people were going hungry on their streets, schools and hospitals had no equipment, houses and bridges were falling down but, as a matter of physiology, they *couldn't* stop.

I am writing this in the shadow of the coronavirus pandemic; China has just announced a drop in new cases but the US is now leading the toll. Whether this means the tide is turning, nobody knows but the omens are certainly not encouraging (actually, it was just the first wave). It has always seemed to me remarkable that we could put so much time and energy into preparing for war but nobody, apart from China and one or two East Asian countries, bothered with even the most rudimentary preparations for this type of disaster. The US still has over 6,000 nuclear weapons and multi-trillion dollar means of dropping those weapons on some duly appointed enemy, but only 62,000 ventilators, one for every 5,000 of the population. Worse, those machines are largely privately-owned, in for-profit hospitals who rent them to whoever pays the price. Rich people, of course, are getting their coronavirus tests, using kits flown in from President Trump's enemy in his trade war, China - duty free, also of course. And all of this has happened because we were all too preoccupied with the battle to dominate each other than to plan for our common welfare.

Australia is no better. We are in the throes of ordering twelve submarines (which have not yet been designed) at a capital cost of $80billion, to be delivered starting in 2035 (assuming no glitches) and concluding in about 2050. Their running costs over their life time will be another $145billion, total $225billion. The reason, we are told, is that we need to be prepared for war, except the only conceivable enemy is our major trading partner, China (even though China has no grievances against or designs on this country: they don't like deserts). Putting aside the fact that we have already spent four years loudly trumpeting what we are going to build and what they are intended to do, and that the Chinese military, who are anything but stupid, will have had about twenty years to devise a means of neutralising our (diesel-powered) submarines (operating at extreme range) with their (nuclear) vessels (operating at their back door), and that other submarines are available now that will do the job for half the price, it should not be forgotten that the catastrophic bushfires which ravaged the nation in the summer of 2019–20 were not unexpected.

For ten years, the political class in Australia had been warned and warned by scientists and fire chiefs that we were heading for an inferno, yet nothing was done. We were too busy spending money on submarines that will be out of date long before the first one is launched than to build firebreaks, or train firefighters, or buy water-bomber aircraft, just to have them ready. Having water bombers sitting ready on a runway is inefficient allocation of capital, they say, whereas having huge sheds full of battle tanks, which will eventually be scrapped without ever having been used, is not.

Similarly with the coronavirus: the researcher who first published the genetic sequence of SARS Covid-19 virus said early in the epidemic that the likelihood of another virus jumping from bats to humans was always known to be very high.

Following the first two coronavirus epidemics (SARS and MERS) and avian and swine influenza, it was not a matter of whether there would be another major zoonotic epidemic, but when it would come and in what form. Had the basic research been done, for a fraction of the cost of operating one submarine for one year, it would have been fairly easy to start producing vaccines within a few months at most. This was known, governments were warned, but they chose to do nothing, because basic biological research or stockpiling ventilators isn't as exciting as watching formations of jets fly overhead or tanks drive past in review - or using the jets and tanks to invade poor nations.

In the human scheme, because domination of each other is so important, we would rather prepare for the faint possibility of war than for the very real and increasing risk of droughts, fires or pandemics. This is because war is so much more exciting and wins votes by appealing to the electorate's worst instincts, the fear of The Other. No country on earth had spare ventilators sitting in a warehouse on the off-chance they may one day be needed because, as they say, storing them is "unnecessary and may cause panic among the citizenry" (as though whipping up fear of attack by screaming hordes of foreign troops doesn't). The safety of the nation takes second place to aggression and domination, because feeling dominant gives lots of politicians, industrialists, financiers and militarists higher blood levels of testosterone. And that is all there is to that.

All talk of bringing democracy to the downtrodden or defending the nation's honour, of protecting our way of life or wars on terrorism, is just that: hollow talk, mere propaganda that conceals the uncontrollable, insensate need to dominate and crush our neighbours. People always need to justify domination, they can always find an excuse for doing what makes them feel good regardless of the cost to others. *The object of power is power.* The politicians and generals will reply: *Si vis pacem, para bellum.* If you want peace, prepare for war. That assumes your neighbour won't misunderstand your motives and will believe you have control over your urge to dominate him, even though all the evidence says you don't. In any event, his innate fear of being dominated forces him to match your build-up, soldier for soldier, weapon for weapon, death for pointless death.

The central problem with domination is that preparing for war exponentially increases the risk of war. If you prepare for war, that is most likely what you will get, whereas preparing for epidemics and bushfires does not increase their risks. But politicians can always find a way of blaming the other side, while generals are never short of imagined dangers for politicians to counter. Politically, domination is an easy sell. It is so much easier to stir up the voters with talk of alien armies threatening our way of life than it is to talk about alien viruses doing the same:

> The right wing politician has less of a distance to go to exploit our tribal fears and hatreds than his opponent, who would engage our better selves (Edgar Doctorow).

Truth is, we can't help ourselves because all humans talk the same language, the language of domination. It has the same appeal to all of us since the mechanism of domination is exactly the same in all humans (albeit somewhat stronger in men). We don't regard it as abnormal to talk of threats by our neighbours: believe it or not, a significant proportion of the Australian electorate actually believe Indonesia is an existential threat to this country. Similarly, even though a shooting war with China would devastate the Australian economy and would probably be over in an hour as a (small) salvo of their hypersonic missiles incinerated our major cities, our politicians are able to sell the fantasy of threatening China with obsolete submarines without anybody stopping to think of its unreality.

Domination controls so much of our thinking that we see it as normal/desirable, and it blinds us to our folly. It is therefore easy for the unscrupulous to convince ordinary people that they need to buy that car, or spend this much on clothes or cosmetic surgery, or that much on weapons, or vote for the war party, all the while neglecting the unfortunate, the downtrodden, the dispossessed, the unfed and unwashed, the unloved and the unlovely. If we don't soon begin to understand how powerful this urge is, if we refuse to see the risks we are laying up for future generations, then I seriously doubt we have a future we would like - or, perhaps, any future at all.

11.4 Free will

Do we have a choice? Is it just a simple matter of saying "Oh well, we need to be a bit more caring so let's dismantle our weapons"? Do we have that choice or are we doomed? In other words, do we have *free will?* The concept of free will says that however I acted one minute ago, I could have acted differently. It is a simple statement but it has major consequences. The Biocognitive Model says we do have free will, and offers a formal mechanism to explain it. To reiterate, a computational process implemented in an active switching device consumes no more energy in computing a correct than an incorrect answer, or no answer at all. As long as there is switching activity, then the outcome is irrelevant to its energy consumption and does not alter the matter-energy balance of the universe.

Any such device that can model future contingencies can therefore predict the outcome of its activities before undertaking them, and can change its parameters accordingly. Once the switching device is running, this consumes no more energy than doing nothing. In the case of our personal switching device, the brain, it is running all the time - the brain doesn't ever switch off. The informational space the brain generates can model the future and can change it before putting it into effect, or even after starting the action.

The capacity to model the future at no metabolic cost confers free will.

This has nothing to do with the brain as a physical thing, and takes place independently of the laws of the material universe, on which determinists base their argument. Remember, this is very fast. Hark back to the cunning butcher birds in Chap **4.5**. In a split second, they can work out where a scrap of food is likely to be and then position themselves to intercept it. If they make a mistake, they can correct for the error in the time the object falls one metre, meaning in 0.45 seconds. In that time, they are flying straight at the ground, fast enough to catch an object travelling at about 16km/hr, and pull out, all without smacking into the floor. If birds can do it, so can we.

Similarly, we can dispel the idea that people can reliably tell the future. Predicting the future means having information about the future. However, there is no means by which an informational state which has not yet been generated can be transmitted back to the past. That is, an informational state can't exist and not exist at the same time. In the biocognitive model, prescience, horoscopes, tarot cards and all ideas of knowing the future are not just physically impossible, they are logically impossible.

However, we are not so rational as we like to believe. We have serious inbuilt cognitive biases, first and foremost being the need to dominate. Because dominating others feels so good, it seems so natural, so much part of life that we don't like to question it. It thus seems that our politicians and leaders in so many fields don't have free will, that they are prisoners of base urges. In a sense, that is true, they are: but only because it brings more votes. It is perfectly feasible that, after World War II, politicians had said "OK folks, that's enough fighting, let's built a better world," but they didn't. The guns never fell silent, the armies never stopped marching, the poor never stopped suffering, because a winner can't stop seeing challenges. Necessarily, because we err on the side of caution, the other side see the winner's triumphal excitement as aggression, and react accordingly. Now our foolishness has brought us to the brink of disaster and we're panicking. But the poor have lived with epidemics and disasters for ever, and who of us cared? We could have done otherwise, but we chose not to.

11.5 Psychiatry

And so, finally, to psychiatry, where, by being written into mental health acts, domination is elevated to the level of law. In 2017 and 2019, the UN Human Rights Commission Special Rapporteur on mental disorder issued reports [1,2] criticising psychiatry for its reliance on a single model of mental disorder, one which assumed the mentally-troubled have no capacity to decide for themselves. In his detailed reports, Lithuanian professor of psychiatry Dainius Puras (b. 1958) urged psychiatrists to pay closer attention to psychosocial contributions to mental disorder, with less reliance on paternalistic models of care:

> 33. Meaningful participation (by patients in mental health policy) has been undermined by entrenched power asymmetries within traditional mental health settings (see A/HRC/35/21). Trust, the bedrock of therapeutic relationships, has been corroded, particularly where coercive and paternalistic practices are prioritized.

His reports were carefully considered, moderate, modest in tone - and attracted a virulent response from mainstream psychiatrists, who felt their corporate interests were threatened. Australian professor and "key opinion leader," Ian Hickie, attacked Puras for daring to suggest there are power asymmetries in mental health practice. Unfortunately, Hickie hadn't done his homework and was absolutely wrong. A person detained in a mental hospital in the state of Queensland has far fewer rights than a prisoner in this state, essentially, none at all. 97% of people appearing before Mental Health Review Tribunals in Qld have no legal representation yet they can be detained by a quasi-judicial procedure using unsworn and hearsay evidence, then locked in isolation, stripped of their clothes, wrestled to the ground and injected without any explanation of the drug, and denied their right to communicate with relatives for as long as the psychiatrist likes. This can and does mean forever, with very limited rights of appeal, all without having broken the law. If that doesn't amount to an asymmetry of power, it isn't clear what would.

Mental health tribunals were established to protect the rights of patients but they have degenerated to the point where they rarely do more than authorise whatever the hospital wants. Because the outcome is so much a foregone conclusion, many patients don't even bother attending their hearings, even if they have been given the documents beforehand. Most don't know they have the right to question the hospital's medical staff and, heavily sedated, befuddled and bewildered, wouldn't know where to start. When it comes to failing to exercise their power of forcing hospitals to make their cases, mental health tribunals are so predictable that they make a rubber stamp look indecisive.

The question we need to ask is: Why does this happen? Whose interests are being served when mentally-troubled people are "classed with infants, imbeciles, and domestic animals"? Bear in mind that mental disorder can happen to anybody. It is the case that those making the decisions on how to "manage" mental disorder have never experienced it. How do we know? Because if they had, they wouldn't be in a position of power. Invariably, they think they have achieved high office by virtue of their innate superiority, especially their superior moral equipment, rather than just by luck, including lucky birth.

As Thomas Szasz (1920–2012) warned, the politicians and psychiatrists and lawyers and police who write and implement mental health laws are all convinced, almost to delusional intensity, that not only do they know everything, that they are not just entitled to make such decisions by virtue of their unimpeachable morality, but they are duty-bound to do so. As one voice, they agree that they are acting for the good of the mentally-disturbed; they feel at ease with their consciences so they never relent, because to do so would be immoral. If holding a person down to jab him with powerful drugs is morally correct, then not doing so is culpable. The problem remains where John Quincy Adams (1767–1848) saw it:

> Power always sincerely, conscientiously, de très bon foi (in very good faith),
> believes itself right. Power always thinks it has a great soul and vast views,
> beyond the comprehension of the weak; and that it is doing God's service
> when it is violating all his laws.

In general medicine, it happens that, despite every effort, some people don't get better. Eventually, they are told: "Sorry, but it looks as though we can't help you. We've tried everything but it hasn't worked so you may as well go home and get on as best you can." In psychiatry, that never happens. A person who says he wants to go home, that the treatment is making him worse or, above all, who resents what the psychiatrists are doing to him, will be given more, not less, "treatment." More drugs, more confinement, more ECT, ever more of the same: treatment without restriction, treatment without accountabilty, treatment without end.

Psychiatrists have a special language for these cases, one which shifts the blame for their failure away from themselves and on to the patient ("a treatment-resistant disorder," "a brittle psychosis"). The parallels between modern psychiatry and historical programs of moral persecution are so close that it becomes difficult to argue against Szasz's claim that, sociologically, they are just variations on the same theme [3].

The problem lies in the human need to dominate, in which respect psychiatrists are no different from any other human. They have exactly the same need to control other people as any other person but... with full legal authority and social approval, they have the means to indulge their urges. To cap it all, because they have sold the idea that they have a scientific understanding of mental disorder, the society never questions them *but* the patients can't. It avails psychiatrists naught to protest that their training has eliminated their need to dominate:

> One has to belong to the intelligentsia to believe things like that: no ordinary man could be such a fool (Orwell again).

The metaphysical problem is that, as it is understood and practiced today, biological psychiatry meshes neatly with the all-but-insatiable human urge to dominate other humans. A mentally-disturbed person is deemed to have a biological disease of the brain. On this basis, he is held to be incapable of making essential decisions for himself, so the state delegates, to the same psychiatrists who have determined his incapacity, responsibility for restoring him to sanity.

If, however, the psychiatrists were wrong in their diagnosis, or if their treatment fails, as treatment often does, then, necessarily, they cannot admit their failure. Inevitably, necessarily, they will fight any attempt to make them admit it, especially when it comes from the patient. This is a trap inherent in the concept of mental incapacity resulting from a biological disturbance of brain function. Psychiatry has had ample opportunity to resolve this conundrum but has never done so because, as Hickie's outburst against Puras showed, they feel too threatened by the loss of power to consider it.

We can look at the parallels in the legal system. The people who arrest somebody for wrongdoing, the police, are not the people who have authority to decide to prosecute. The people who decide to prosecute are not the people who determine guilt. That rests with the jury, who have no interests in common with the police and may even dislike them. Finally, those who determine guilt do not pass sentence. It would not be good if police were also prosecutors, judges and juries; we call that a police state.

But, in the case of mental disorder, psychiatrists are in control every step of the way. Nobody, least of all themselves, can tell when they cross the line from the genuine wish to help a distressed person to tormenting that person because he refuses to submit to their will. Too many psychiatrists appear incapable of admitting they may be wrong, that they don't have a model of mental disorder, and that their "treatments" may be doing more harm than good. Not only do psychiatrists have a lot to hide, but they have the legal means to hide it. Only they can reveal it but, because their incomes depend on not revealing it, they remain silent. And by bestowing such untrammelled power to a profession which has so much in common with cults, the state is complicit in their cover-ups.

The whole concept of enforced treatment is based on the unproven assumption that the brains of mentally-troubled people are diseased, so *ipso facto,* they cannot make valid decisions for themselves. But if that assumption is false, just because there is no brain disease, meaning the whole biological program in psychiatry is just wishful thinking, what then is the justification for holding people against their will for decades and pumping them full of drugs that shorten life?

As for enforced treatment, it is a little-known fact that although most psychiatrists believe the incidence of, say, bipolar disorder is up to 15% of the population, and anybody who has the diagnosis must be drugged, even against his will if necessary, it is extremely rare for psychiatrists themselves to be given the diagnosis. That is, simply by training in psychiatry, they seem to gain protection from what they claim to be a genetic disorder. This demands explanation. I mentioned this to a very experienced psychiatrist who sees a lot of doctors for the Medical Board and who treats adolescents and families in therapy. "Oh," came the breezy reply, "you'll never see a psychiatrist take their own drugs, or go into a mental hospital, or get ECT. But what you do see is that they manage to get their relatives on drugs, especially their children."

Finally, it is worth noting that medical students don't like psychiatry. All around the world, there is a growing shortage of young medical graduates entering psychiatric training. When asked why, students say it is boring and non-scientific. The students are correct:

> The system filters out the thoughtful and replaces them with the faithful. When everybody is thinking the same thing, nobody is thinking at all.

Academic psychiatrists have achieved something which, when I started psychiatry, I would not have thought possible: they have managed to make psychiatry boring. The problem is that these days, conformity to the prevailing ethos, meaning mindless reductionism, is valued over critical intelligence. I cannot see that as anything other than a very great crime. Even though it doesn't last, students are entitled to a sense of excitement.

11.6 Treatment of mental disorder

In two paragraphs, treatment of mental disorder is based in finding the causes of symptoms, *of understanding symptoms but not suppressing them.* If symptoms are suppressed this week, using drugs and ECT and so on, they will pop up again next week, but worse because of side effects of the treatment. Of course, psychiatrists don't believe their treatment has side effects, anything that goes wrong, such as akathisia, obesity, confusion, loss of libido, addiction, suicidal ideas etc, is either the patient's fault (obesity), not worth worrying about (impotence), not true (addiction), or signs of further mental disorder and a reason to give more drugs etc (all the rest, especially akathisia).

Mental symptoms have mental causes, which can only be uncovered by careful investigation of the patient's recent life and his personality. That is because *symptoms must be seen in their causative context,* including early life experiences (which shaped the personality) and recent events, which exposed the personality weaknesses. All of this dictates that the psychiatrist will devote a considerable amount of time, energy and craft to making contact with the patient on a level he can understand and accept, and then exploring his life until the causes of his distress become clear. A disturbed informational state, which is what a mental disorder *is*, needs to be untangled. That means talking *with* the patient, not *at* the patient. Thus, treatment in psychiatry is psychological, not biological, talk therapy, not drug therapy or convulsive therapy. Over the past 150 years, a biological psychiatry has failed to prove itself, so it is now time to move on.

11.7 An afterthought on religion.

"What about religion?" This question was put to me by a non-medical colleague who keeps a sharp eye on psychiatry. "What does your theory say about the concept of, say, immortality?" Good question. The answer is that, in the bio-cognitive model for psychiatry, the functioning, intact, healthy brain is necessary for the emergence of the mind. There can be no disembodied information and therefore no ghosts or free-ranging spirits. At the point of death, when all brain activity ceases, the emergent mind will also cease to exist. All awareness of a self will cease, for all time. That would seem to be encouraging to the atheist side of the debate but, before they start cheering, they should consider some other consequences of this model.

There is no a priori reason to suppose that emergent mentality is restricted to biological (carbon-based) data processing systems. That is, silicon-based computers may eventually be able to see red, experience pain and laugh at jokes - or get angry. If, at the point of death, the entire informational content of a person's brain were uploaded to a suitable, non-biological, data processing system, then the mind would not cease to exist. Recreated in facsimile in the new system, it could last forever. I am not saying this happens, I am saying only that it is a logical possibility. How could this be done? By some vastly superior technology that is far beyond our dreams at present - perhaps even as far as 2020 technology is from 1820 technology. As Arthur Clarke said, Any sufficiently advanced technology is indistinguishable from magic.

That's fine, but what about God? If there is no disembodied information, how does she exist as a spirit? That I don't know, but I do know that the observable universe which we inhabit is but a small part of the total matter-energy content of the universe. About 27% of the universe is dark matter and 68% is dark energy, leaving only 5% for our tangible universe. If, as rationalists suppose, mental properties arose on this planet through mindless processes of evolution acting over aeons, there is no reason to conclude that the same thing could not have happened in the dark universe, although it wouldn't be dark to its residents. There is also no reason to suppose their technology would be inferior to ours, so whatever they do would most likely appear to be magic to us. Indeed, compared with us, they would seem god-like.

This is not an attempt to convert all religious people to the idea that their divinity is more prosaic than previously believed, nor even to start a new religion (even though it would probably be more profitable than writing abstruse books). Rather, it says to the rowdy group of publicity-minded atheists: Be careful. Every argument you use to support the notion of the rational emergence of life on earth can be turned and used against you. As for people who argue that life didn't emerge on earth but was seeded from interstellar space, also wrong. The information may have come from elsewhere (I doubt it) but it would not have been effective unless it were taken up by fully-functioning cells. Anyway, the chemicals were local.

11.8 To build a new reality

To return to the quote by Buckminster Fuller on the frontispiece,

> You never change something by fighting the existing reality. To change something, build a new model that makes the existing model obsolete.

For many years, I have been contending with the existing reality of psychiatry, using arguments that have never been refuted but, strangely enough, the old psychiatry is still there, it hasn't changed or gone away. What is its existing reality? Almost the entire practice of modern psychiatry is built on the concept of reductionism, that mental disorder reduces to a physical disorder of the brain. Don't worry that this has never been established, that no psychiatrist has ever written a proper account of what the idea entails or an objective defence: it is the Received Truth that trainees must accept without question if they wish to graduate. We are therefore compelled to ask: What are the forces holding this destructive travesty in place?

A few say it remains in place because it is based in a "biomedical model" but they never specify what it models. Is it a model of normal mental life, or specifically of mental disorder? Does it account for personality disorder or even lead to a model of normal personality? None of this is known because, once again, nobody has published anything that could constitute a "biomedical model."

Other influential psychiatrists endorse as psychiatry's guiding light something called the "biopsychosocial model," which they attribute to George Engel (1913-99), a gastroenterologist of Rochester, NY. This was widely accepted as the definitive statement of psychiatry's claim to be a unique medical specialty. Melbourne psychiatrist, Bruce Singh, who knew Engel well enough to visit him at home in his twilight years, conceded his mentor was "driven by a narcissistic belief in his own 'specialness'" and saw himself as a "medical Darwin." Singh, for one, was in no doubt as to its value, to psychiatry and to medicine as a whole: "What no one can deny is that (Engel left) a towering edifice …."

This is a little strange as, in 1998, I showed that Engel's model didn't exist, that he never actually wrote it [4]. It is now clear that Engel had made a fundamental mistake [5]. He thought naming his model would also define it, but it is not possible to nominate an entity and define it in the same illocutionary act. He never got around to writing an integrative model of mind, body and society. However, so desperate were psychiatrists for a model, any model, that would lift them to the same level as the rest of medicine, that they overlooked this slight failing. Singh's "towering edifice" was an illusion, nothing more than mutually-reinforced self-deception, a tower of bullshit, as defined by Princeton philosopher, Harry Frankfurt [6].

In the absence of a formal model of mental disorder, psychiatry has degenerated into an ideology. Hence this small volume, whose goal is to render that ideology obsolete. This work represents the culmination of over forty years study and research. Whatever its shortcomings, the biocognitive model for psychiatry is the first serious attempt at a formal model of mental disorder based in an articulated theory of mind. At this stage of theory development in psychiatry, whether it is correct or not hardly matters - as far as theories or models for psychiatry go, it has no competition.

Because it directly challenges the prevailing approach, challenges their domination, I don't expect my work to meet a rapturous response from the people it aims to put out of a job. So back to the quetion above: What are the forces holding this destructive travesty in place? We can answer that with an alliteration: Commerce, conceit and connections. The influence of drug companies needs no elaboration. The conceit and arrogance of academic psychiatrists, who have built "a towering edifice" of intellectual deceit, is a major force but they hold this in place by carefully wrought political connections and backroom dealing [7,8].

My goal is therefore to appeal to the new generation of psychiatrists. The older generations are a lost cause, hopelessly compromised by their unthinking embrace of biological reductionism. Whether the biocognitive model succeeds or fails depends on whether today's students are prepared to think critically about their field, and not just fall into line with whatever the "key opinion leaders" determine they should memorise. That is, students and trainees must exercise their right to criticise the establishment, to challenge their dominance. Science isn't about opinions, it's about what can survive a barrage of criticism, especially self-criticism, which psychiatry suppresses. Whether this model survives, and in what form, time will tell, but it stands as the most direct challenge to modern psychiatry in many years.

References

[1] UN Human Rights Council (2017) Report of the Special Rapporteur on the right of everyone to the enjoyment of the highest attainable standard of physical and mental health. Available at: https://www.refworld.org/docid/593947e14.html (accessed November 10th 2019).

[2] UN Human Rights Council (2019). Report of the Special Rapporteur on the right of everyone to the enjoyment of the highest attainable standard of physical and mental health. (2019) UNHRC Document A/HRC/41/34, at: https://documents-dds-ny.un.org/doc/UNDOC/GEN/G19/105/97/PDF/G1910597.pdf?OpenElement Accessed November 10th 2019.

[3] Szasz TS (1974). *The Myth of Mental Illness: Foundations of a Theory of Personal Conduct.* Revised Edition. New York: Harper and Row (Perennial Library).

[4] McLaren N (1998). A critical review of the biopsychosocial model. *Australian and New Zealand Journal of Psychiatry.* 32: 86–92. Revised version: McLaren N (2010). A life of its own: the strange case of the biopsychosocial model. Chapter 7 in *Humanizing Psychiatrists: Toward a Humane Psychiatry.* Ann Arbor, Mi.: Future Psychiatry Press.

[5] McLaren N (2020). The Biopsychosocial Model: the end of a reign of error. *Ethical Human Psychology and Psychiatry.* 22: 71–82.

[6] Frankfurt H (1986). On Bullshit. *Raritan Quarterly Review* 6, No. 2 (Fall 1986).

[7] Whitaker R, Cosgrove L (2015). *Psychiatry Under the Influence: Institutional Corruption, Social Injury, and Prescriptions for Reform.* New York: Palgrave MacMillan.

[8] Gotzsche P (2015). *Deadly Psychiatry and Organised Denial.* London: Artpeople.

Index

References to figures are indicated in *italics* and references to tables in **bold**. References to footnotes consist of the page number followed by the letter 'n' followed by the number of the note.

Printed in the United States
by Baker & Taylor Publisher Services